Rex The Lion
Wears a Mask

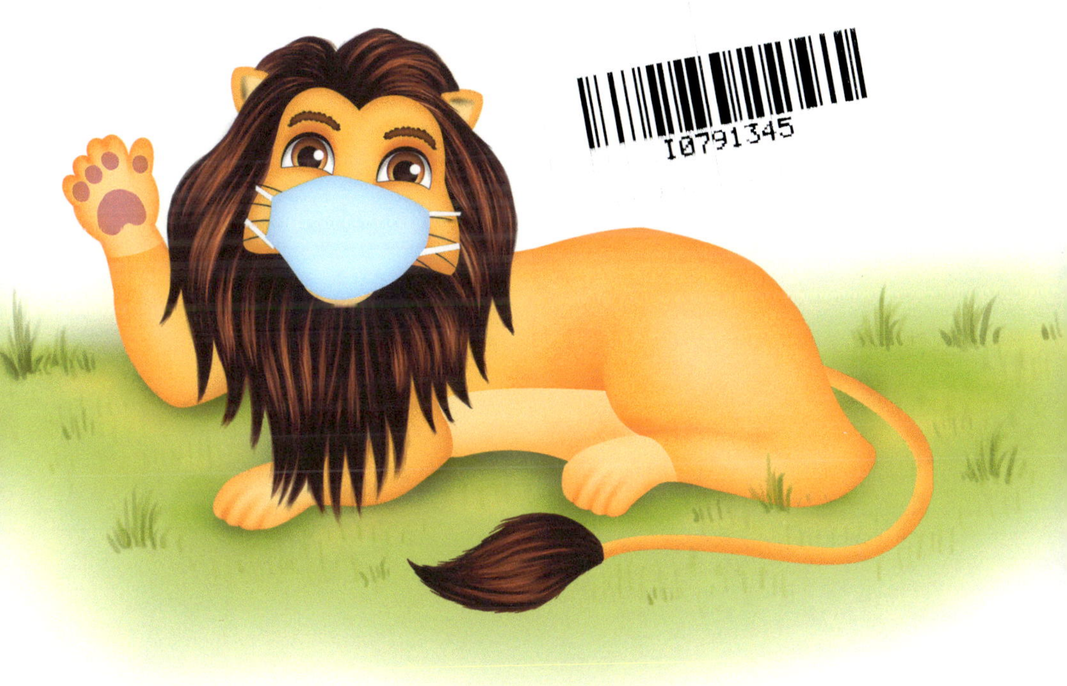

By : Elon Ram

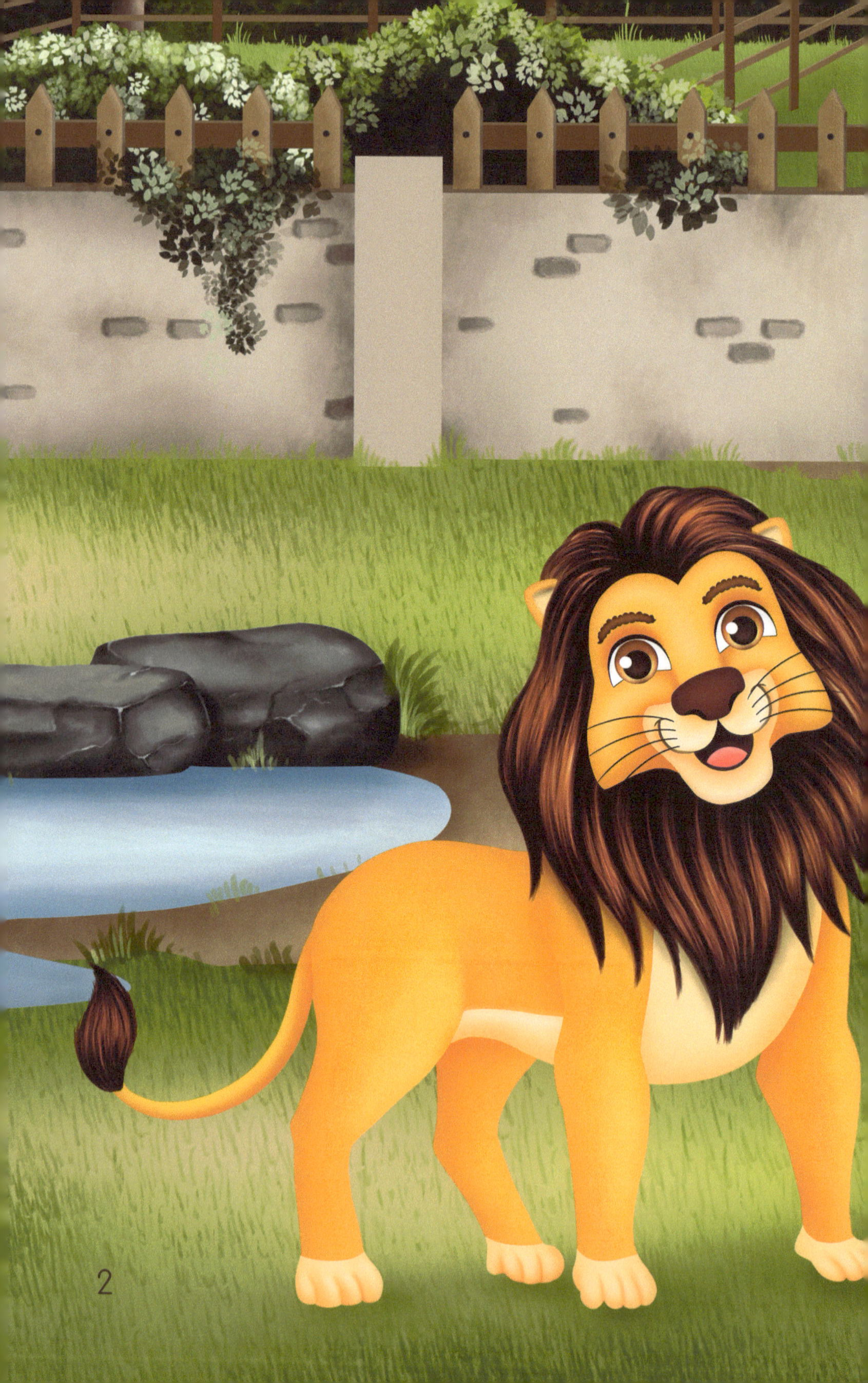

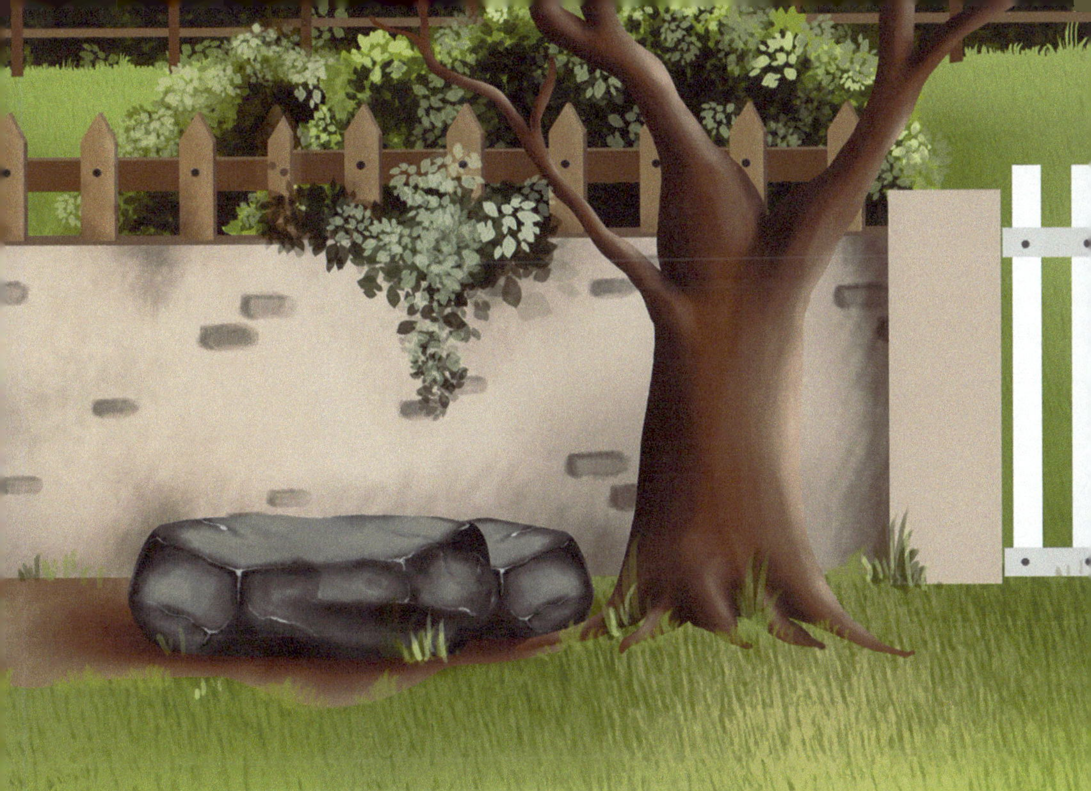

Rex the lion was a
handsome fellow,
with a fluffy mane that was
brown and yellow.

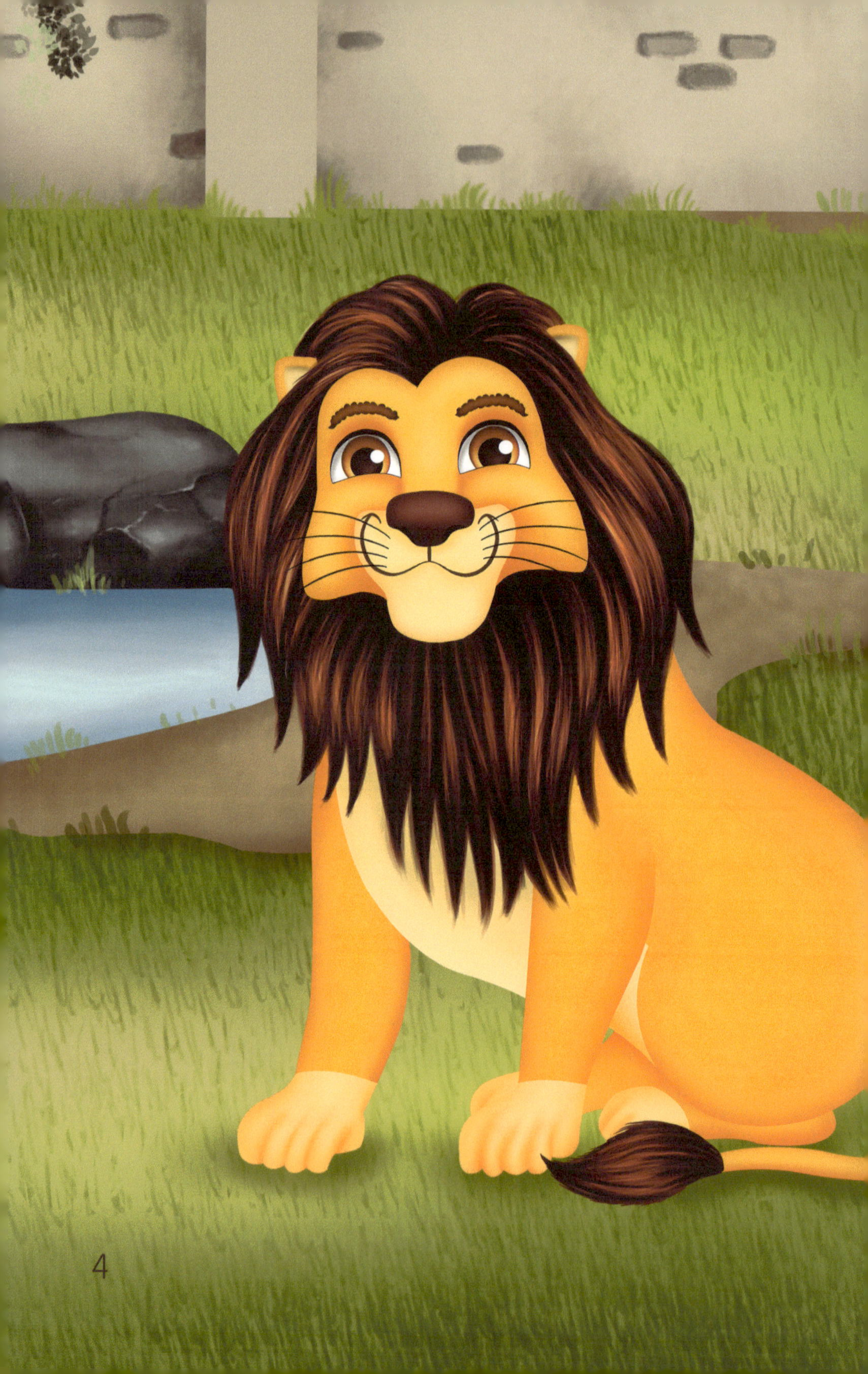

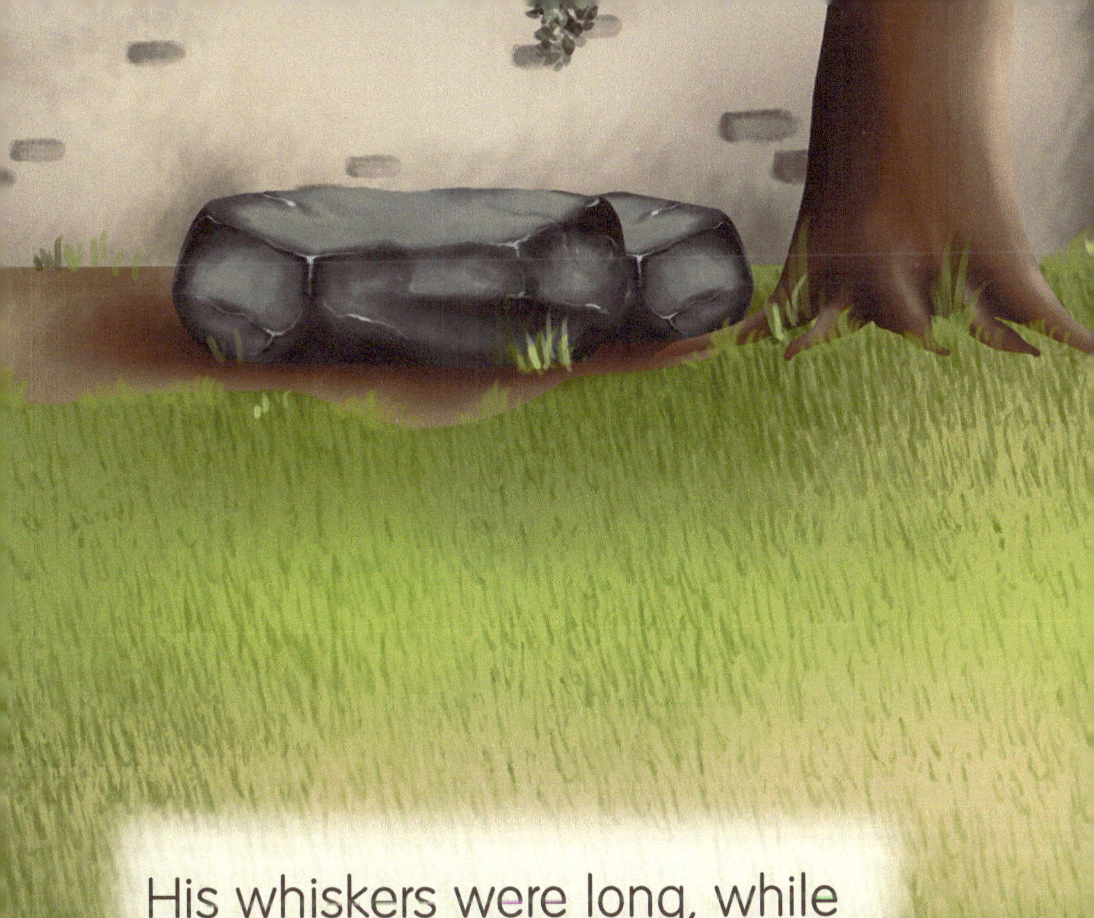

His whiskers were long, while **his ears were short** and his eyes were of the **kindest sort.**

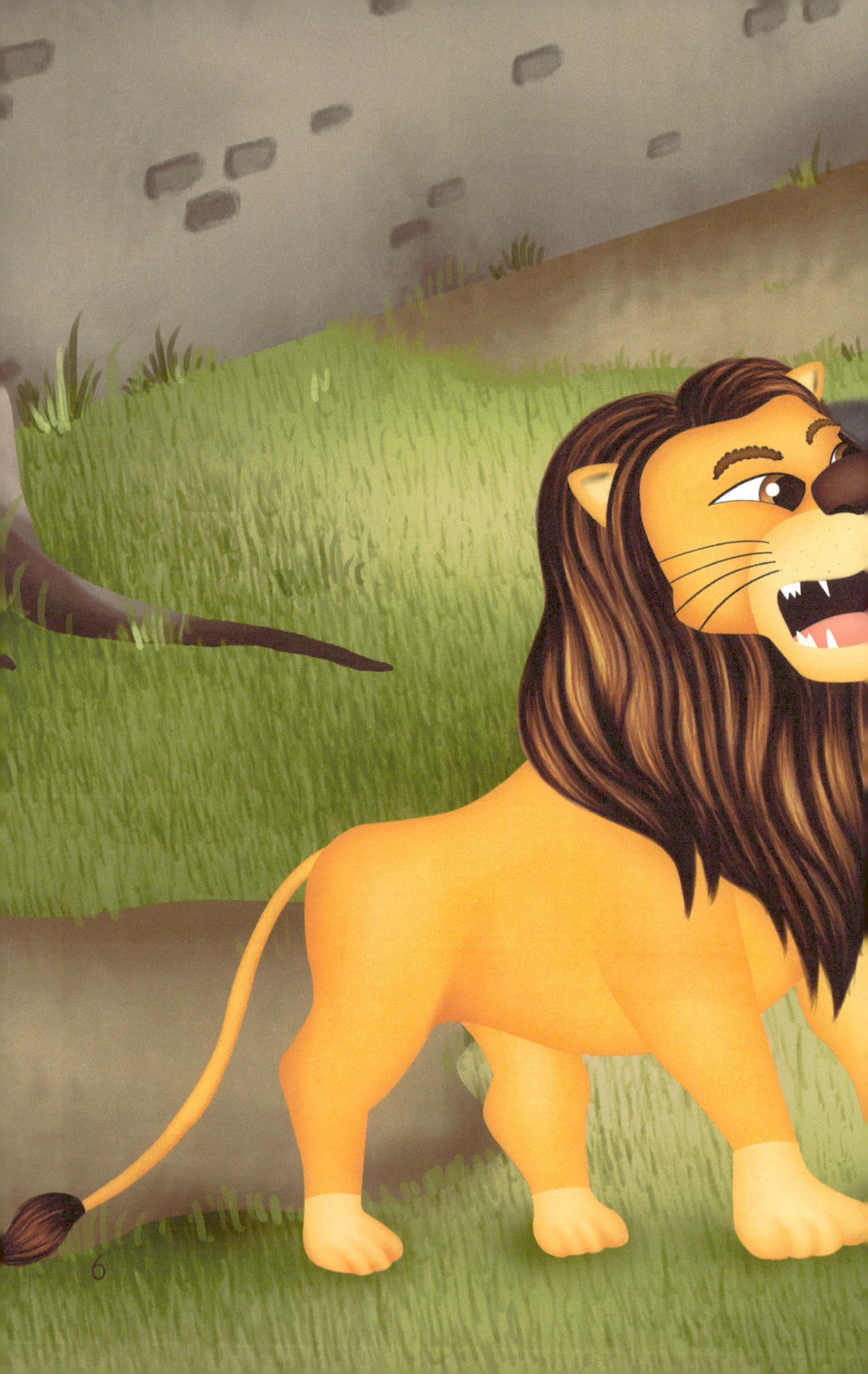

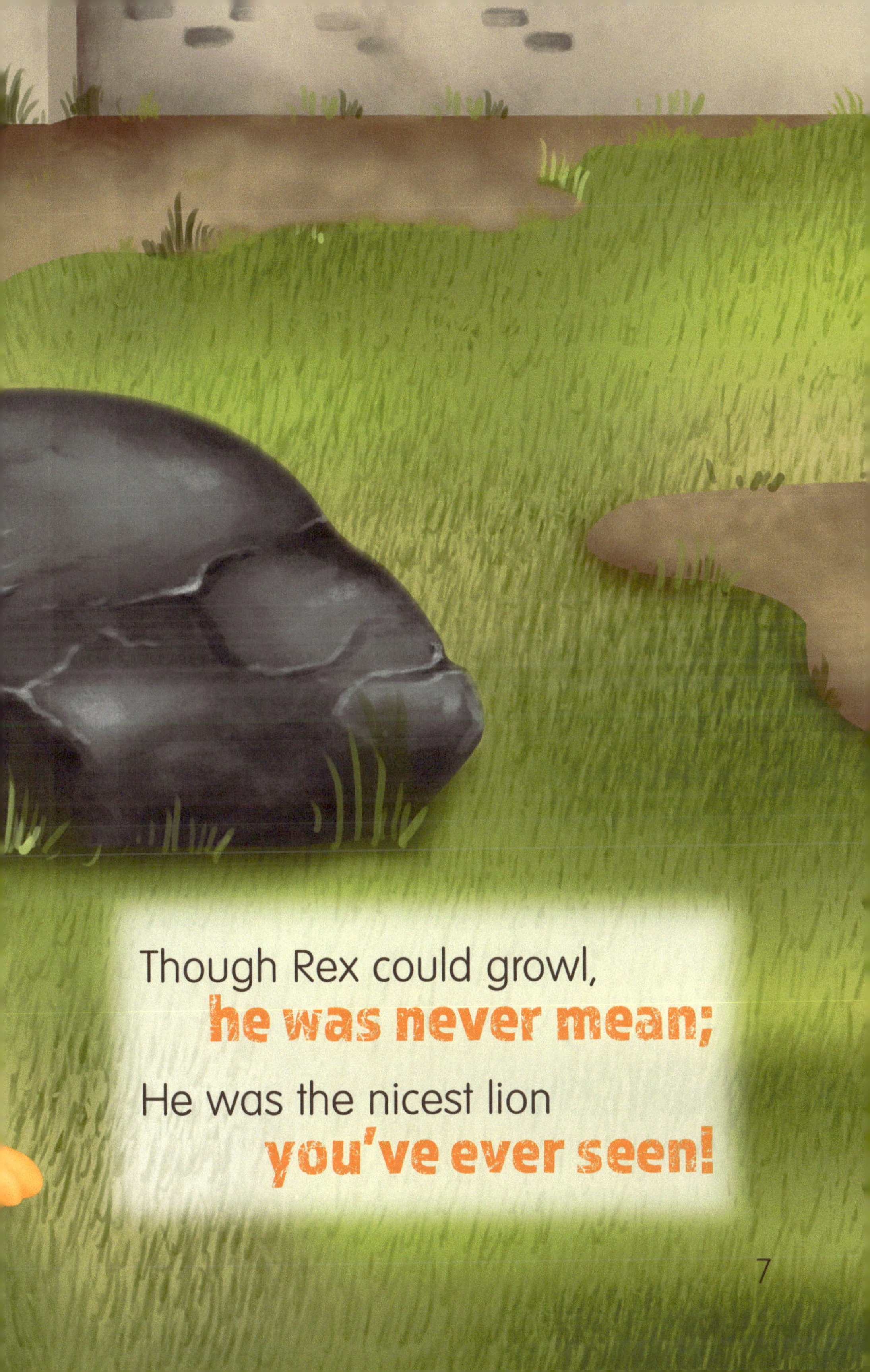
Though Rex could growl,
he was never mean;
He was the nicest lion
you've ever seen!

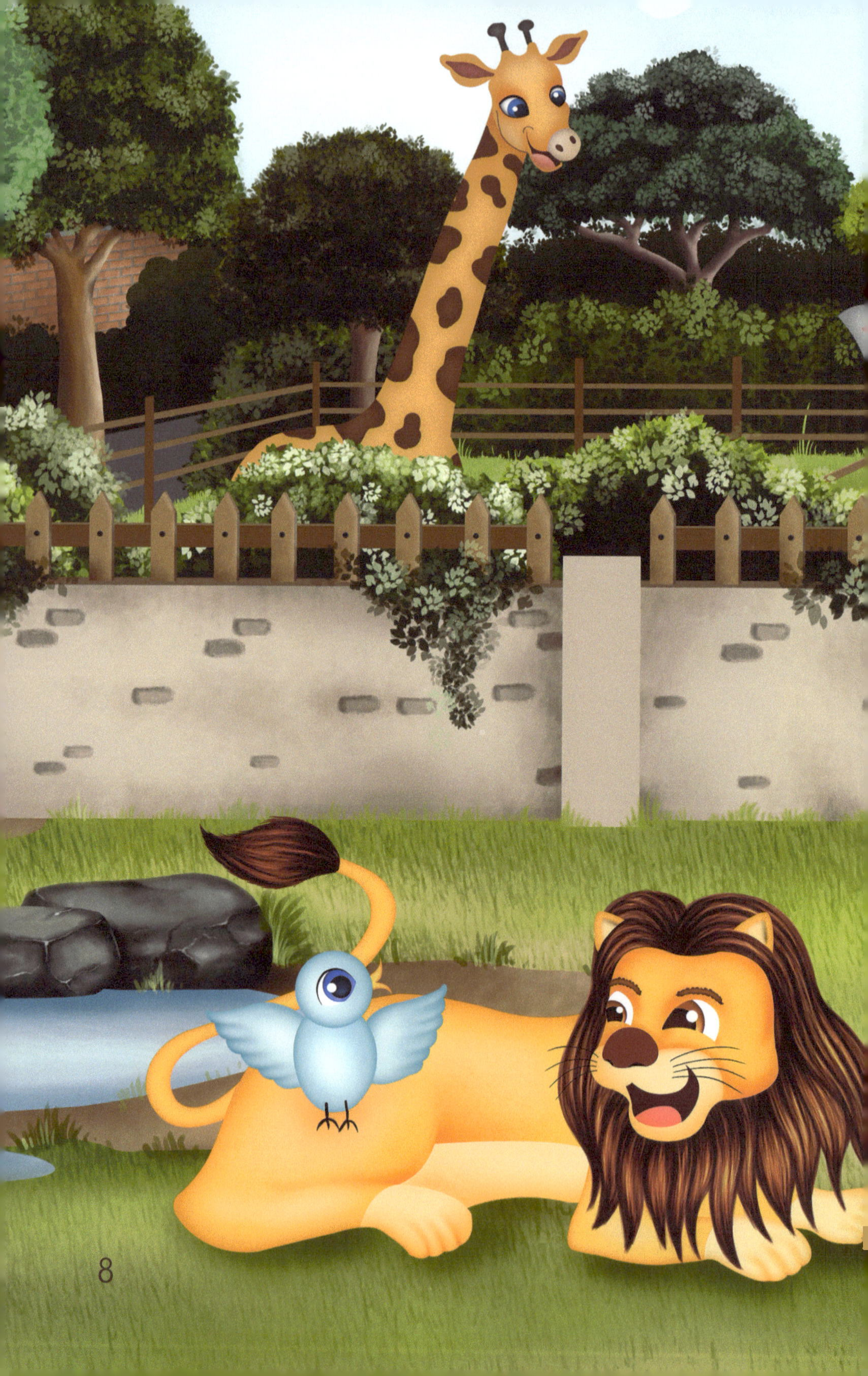

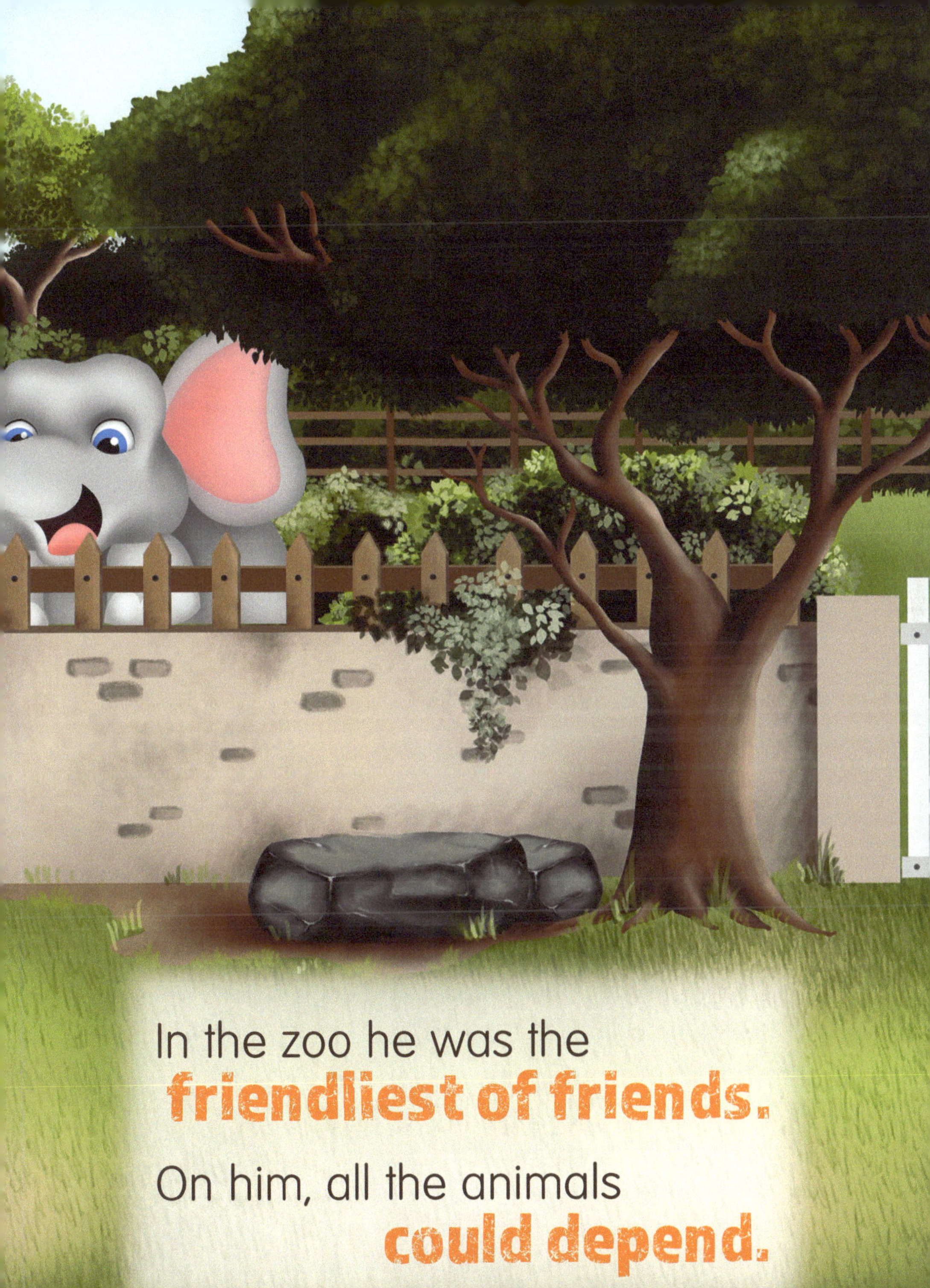

In the zoo he was the
friendliest of friends.

On him, all the animals
could depend.

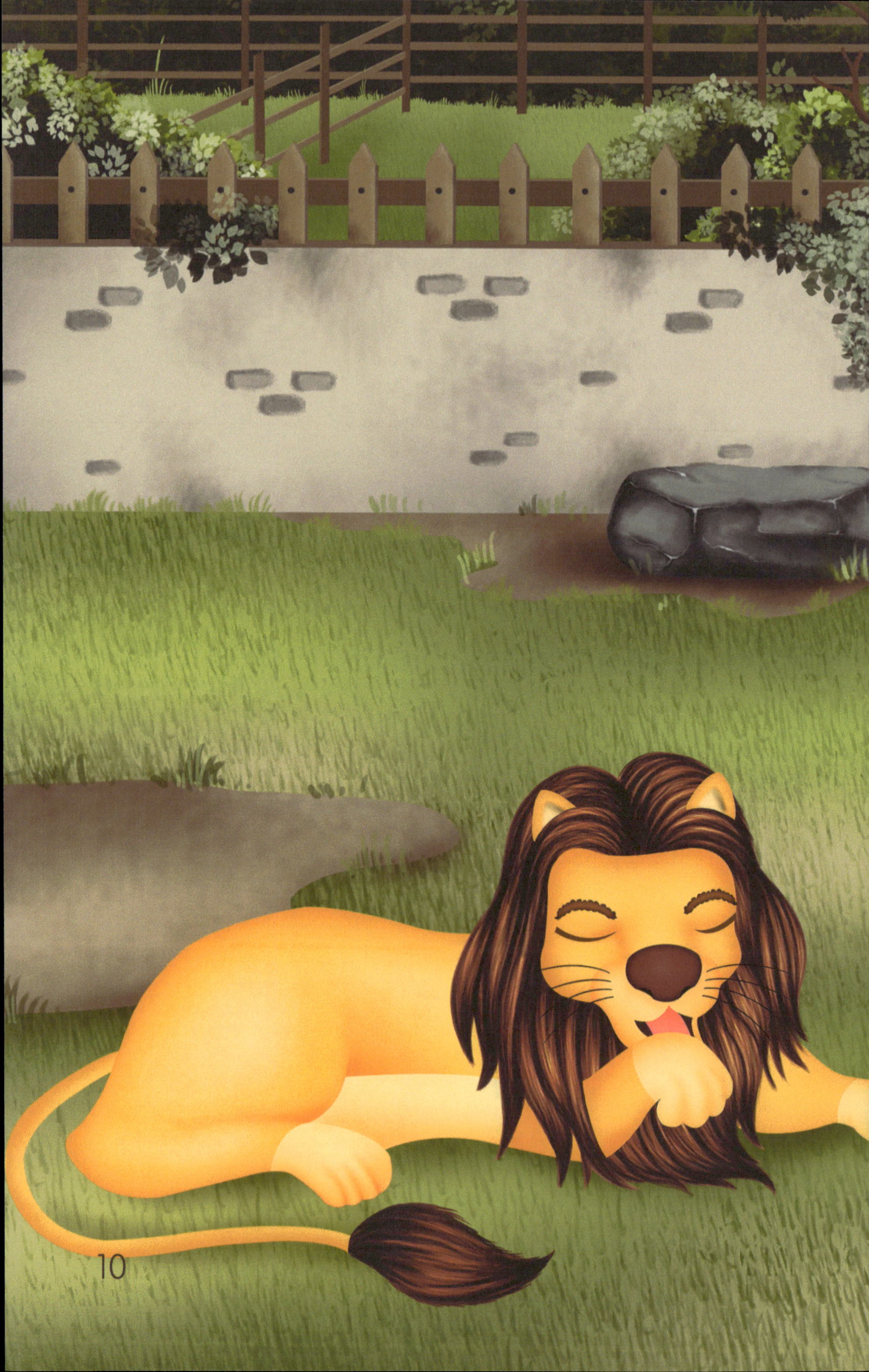

10

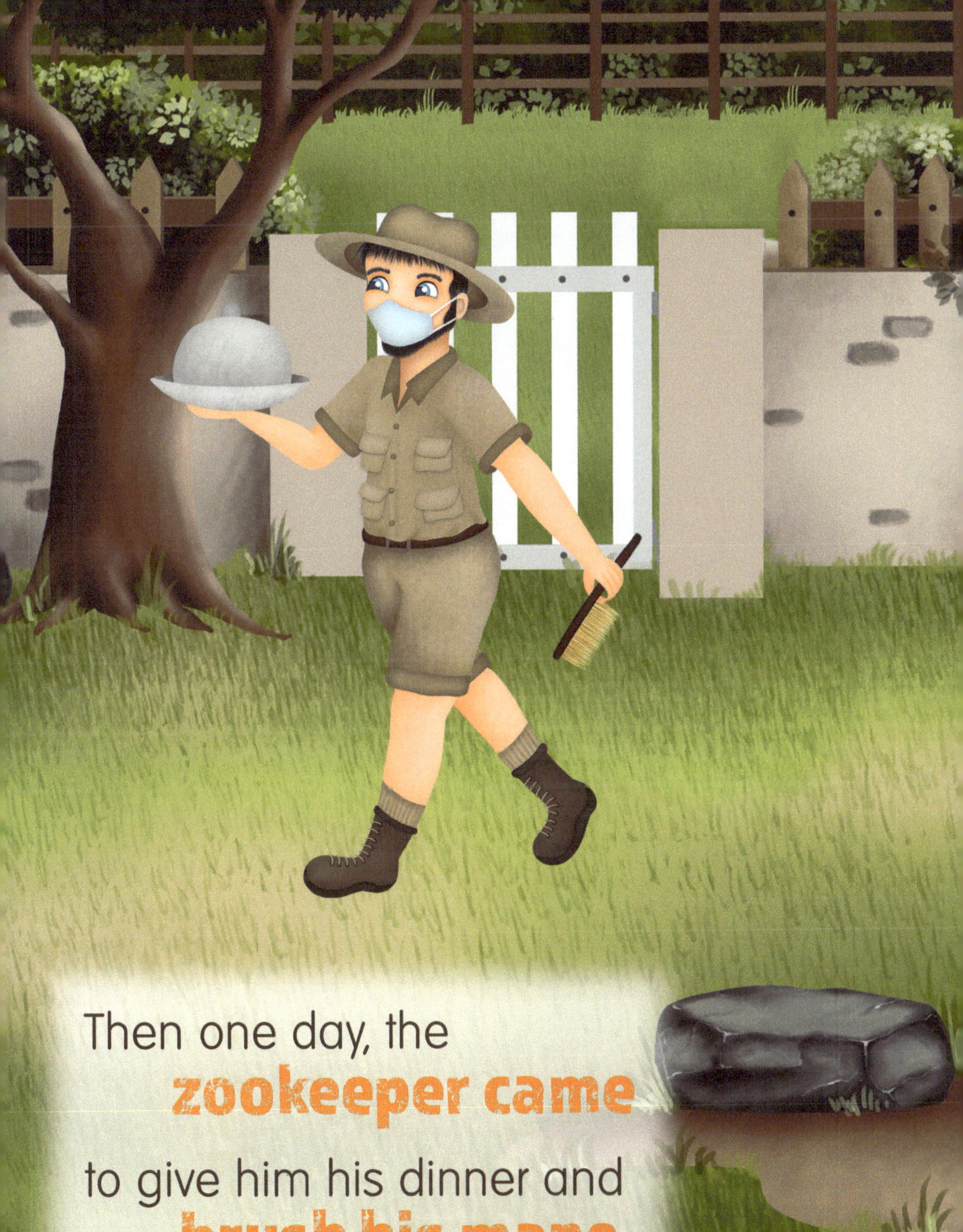

Then one day, the
zookeeper came
to give him his dinner and
brush his mane.

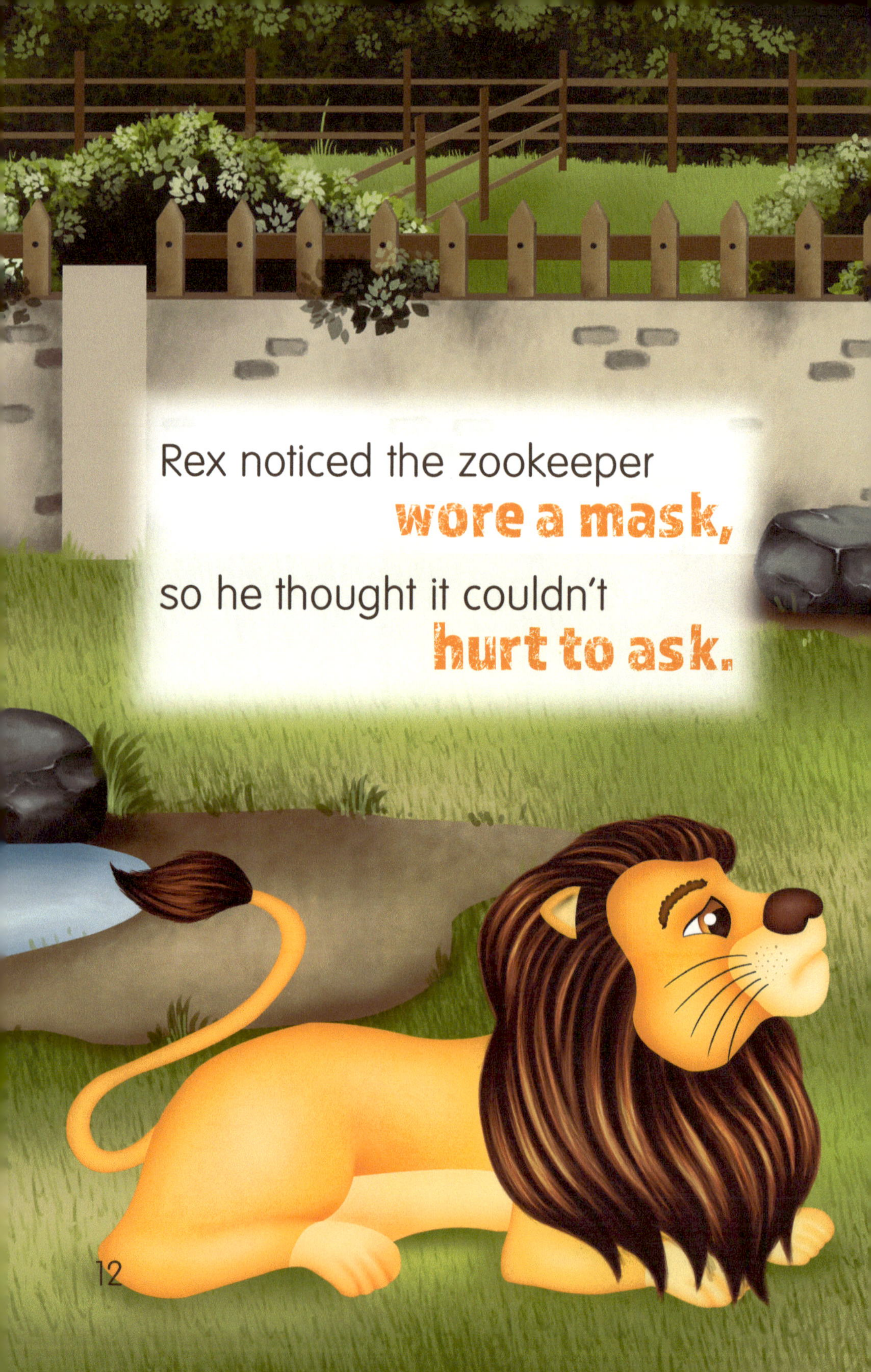

Rex noticed the zookeeper **wore a mask,** so he thought it couldn't **hurt to ask.**

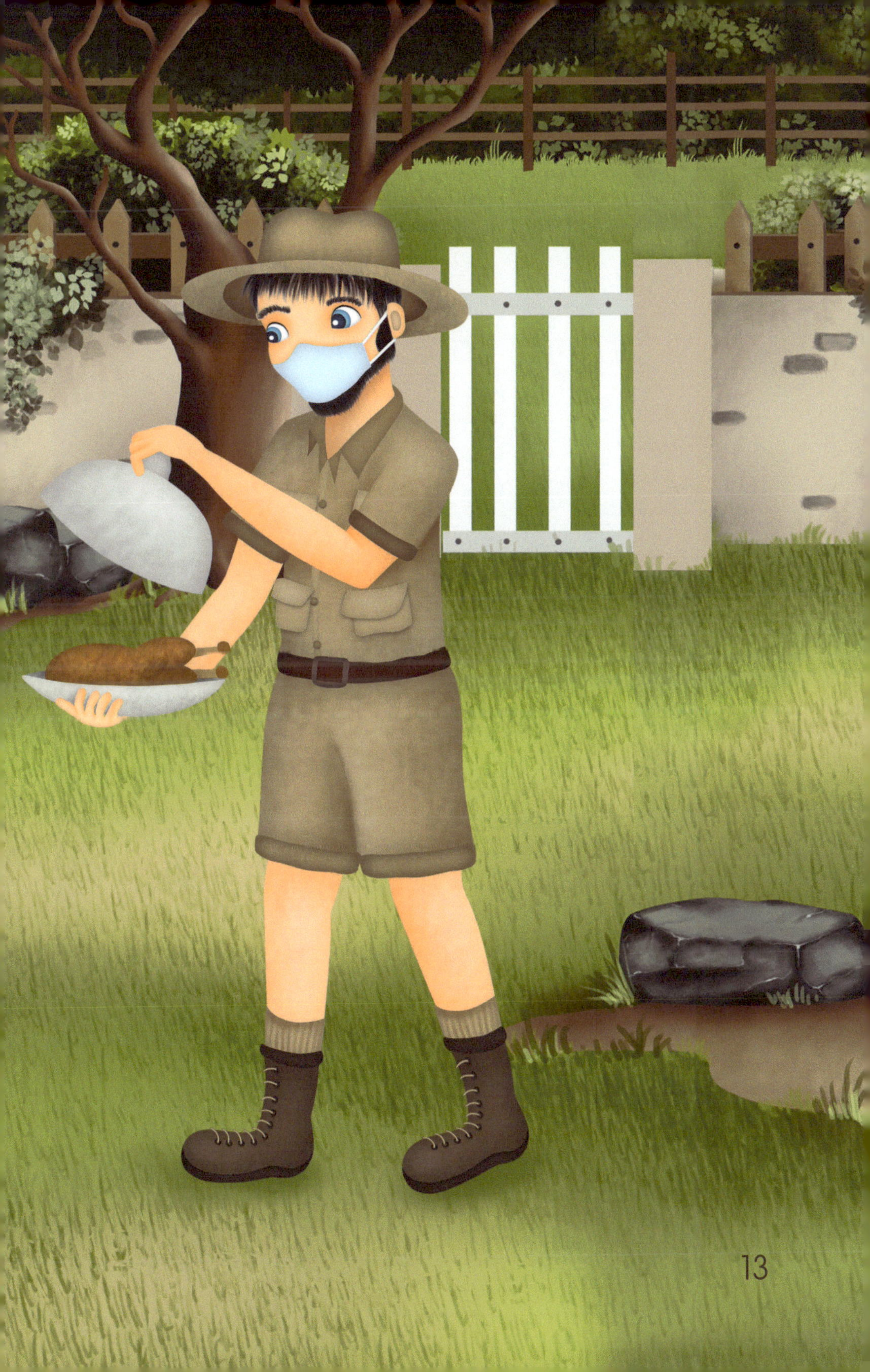

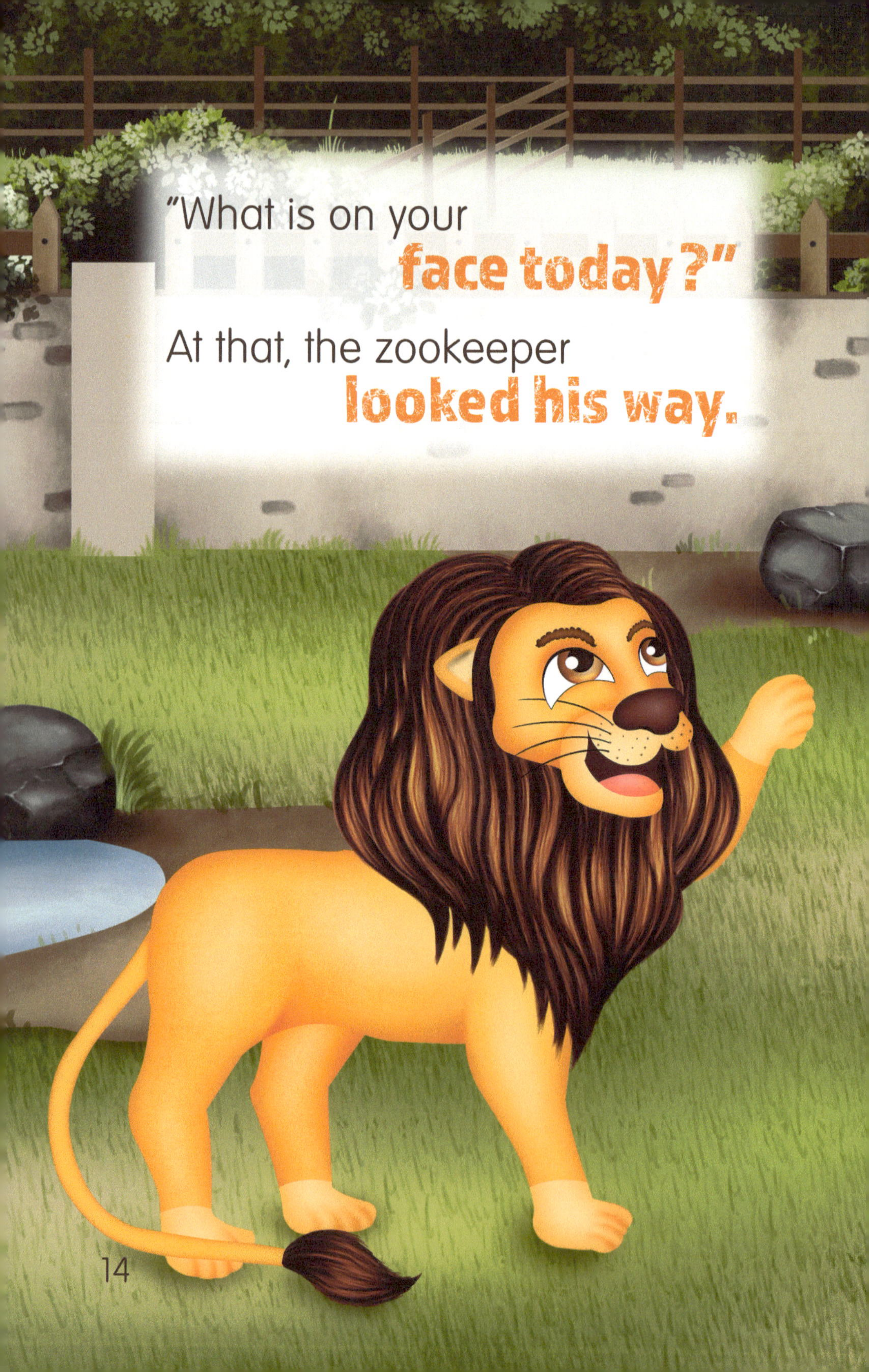

"What is on your face today?"
At that, the zookeeper looked his way.
14

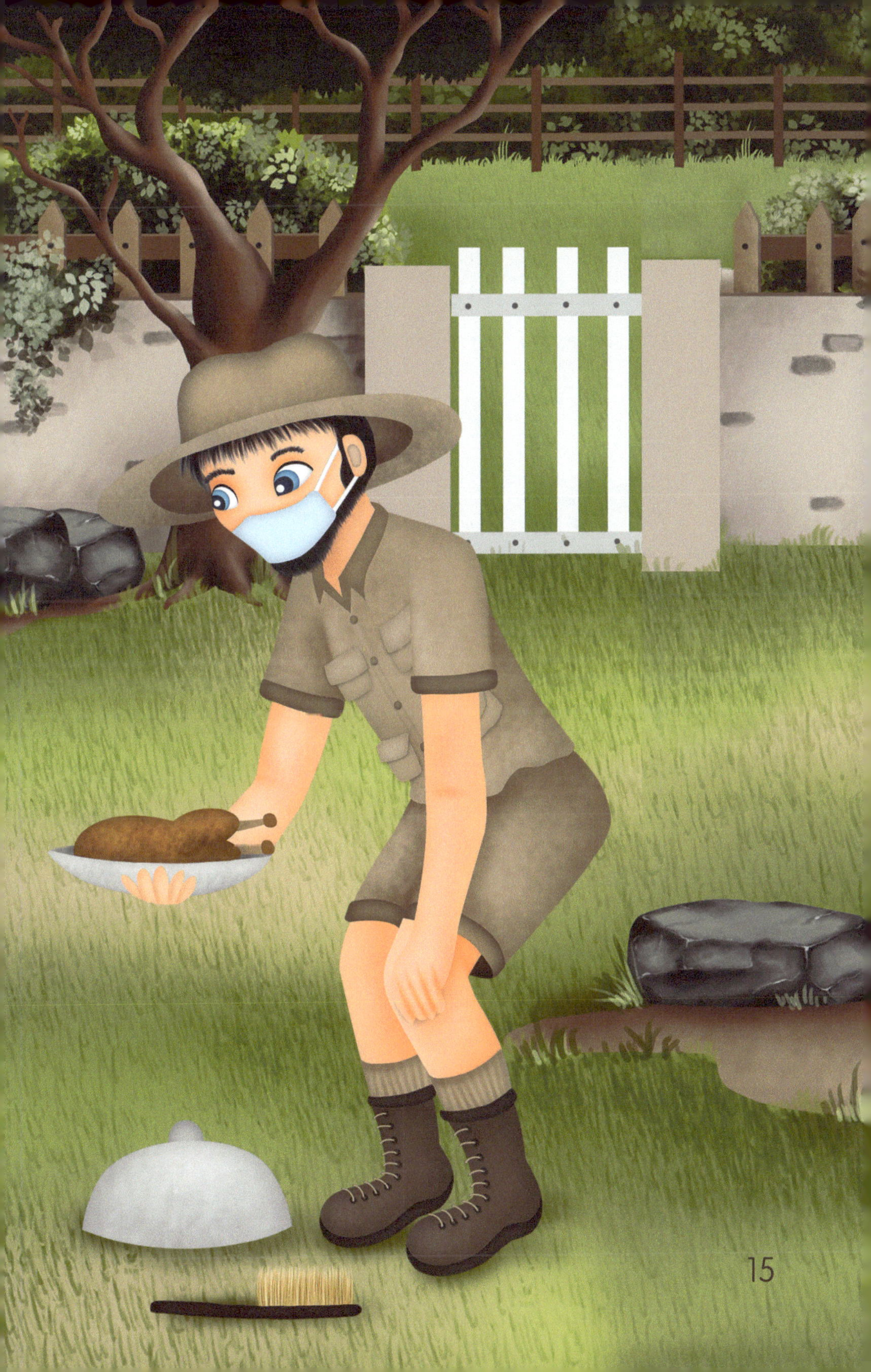

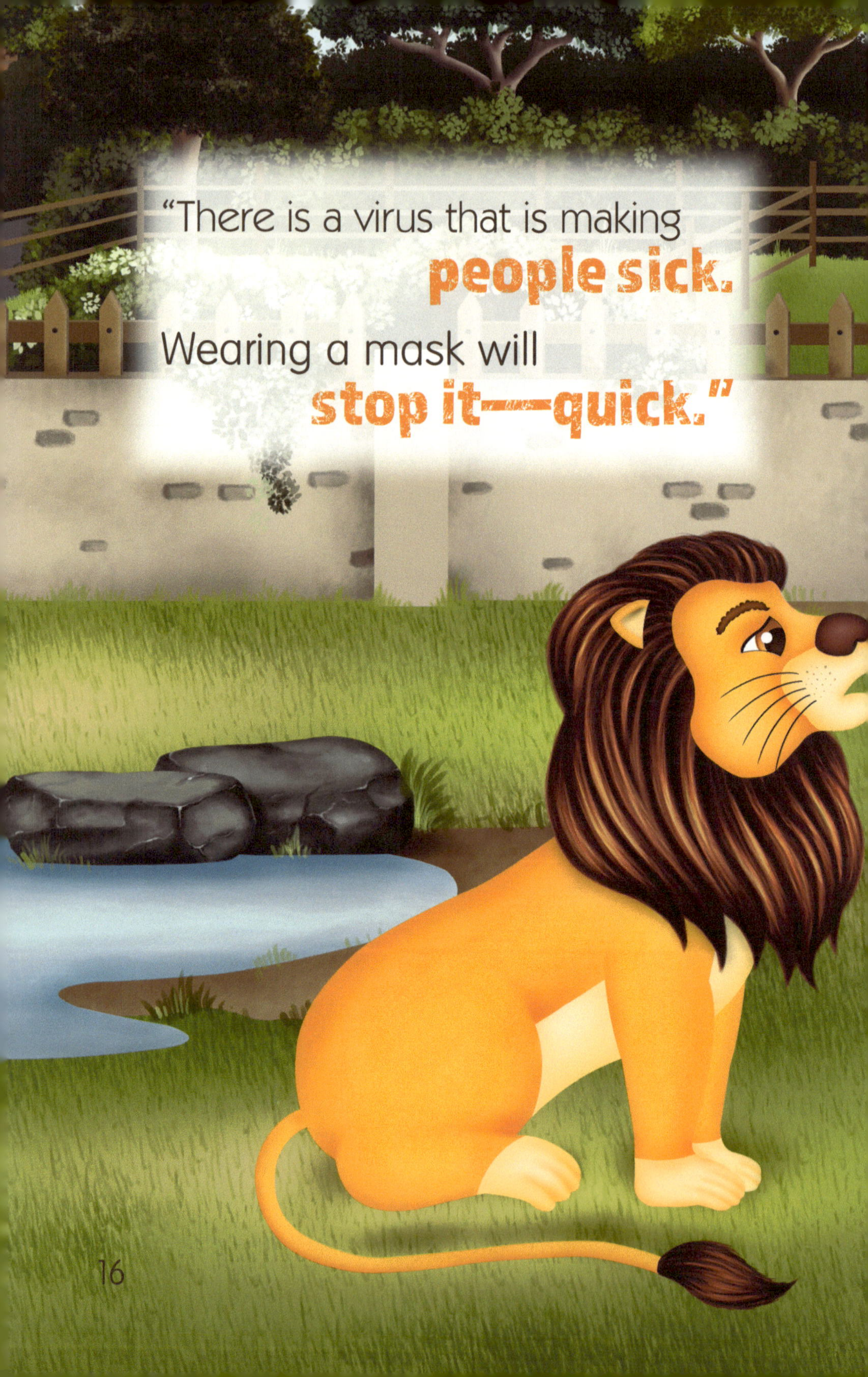

"There is a virus that is making people sick.
Wearing a mask will stop it—quick."

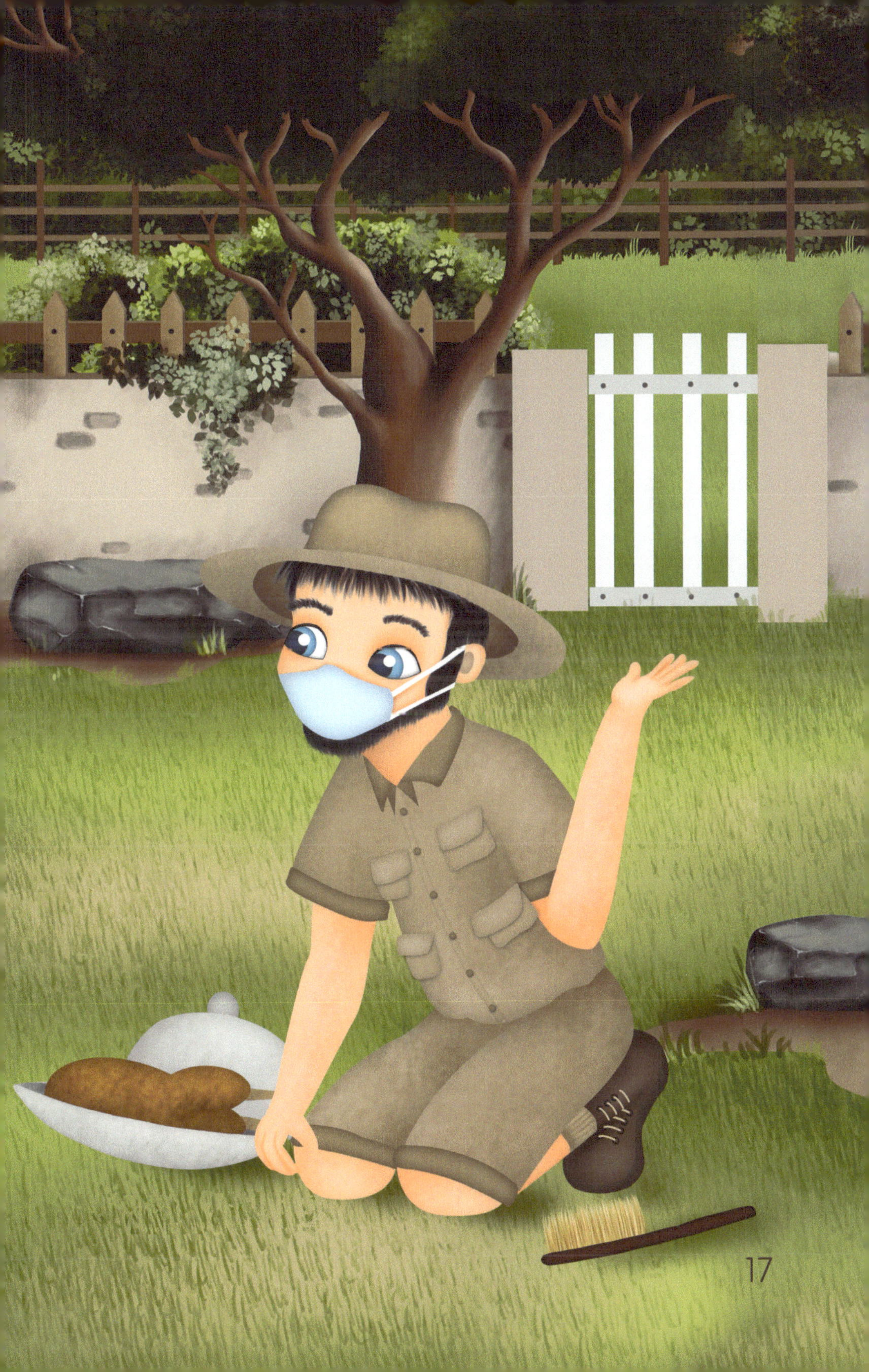

Then Rex asked,
"Can I wear one, too?"
The zookeeper nodded.
"I have one for you!"

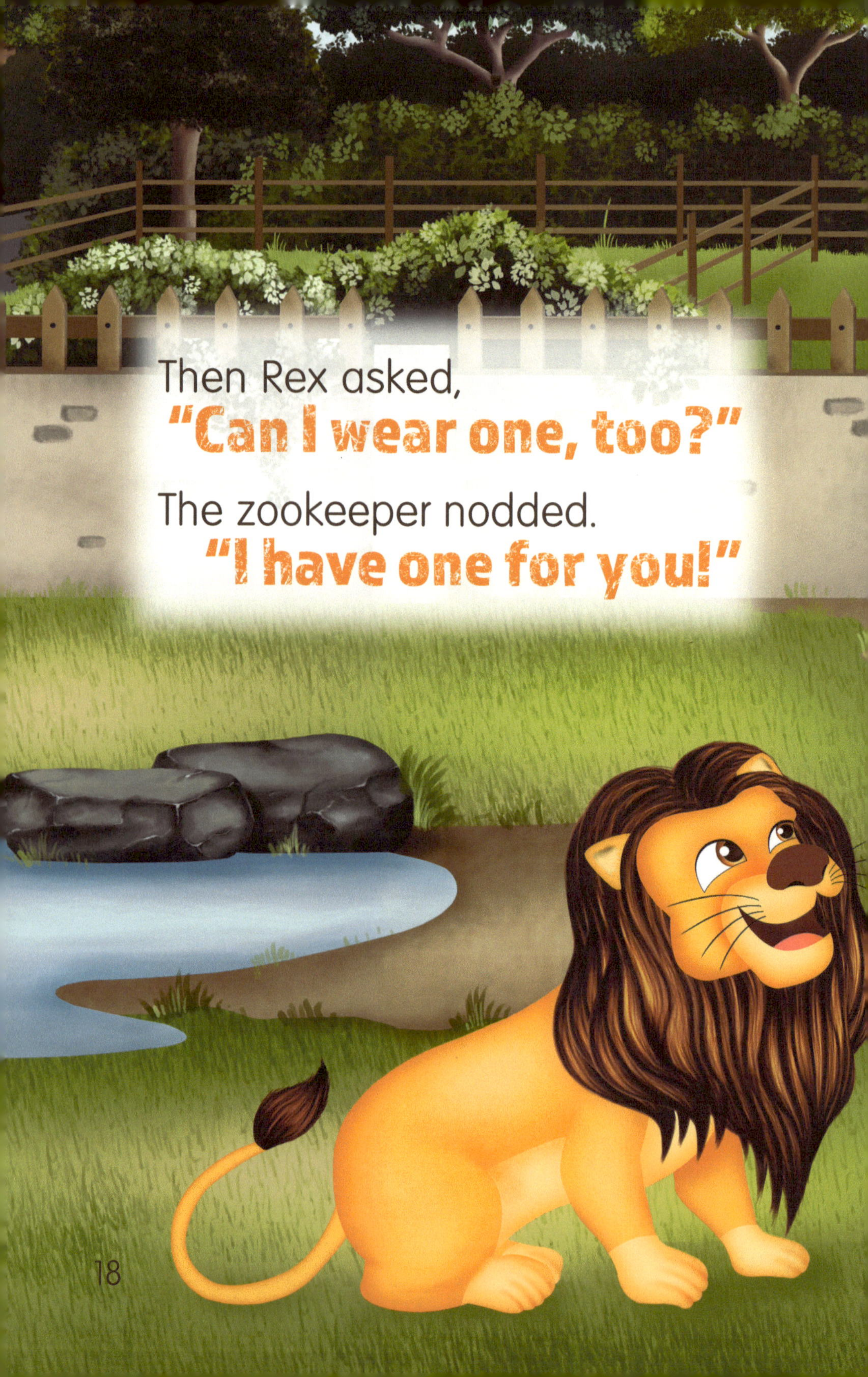

18

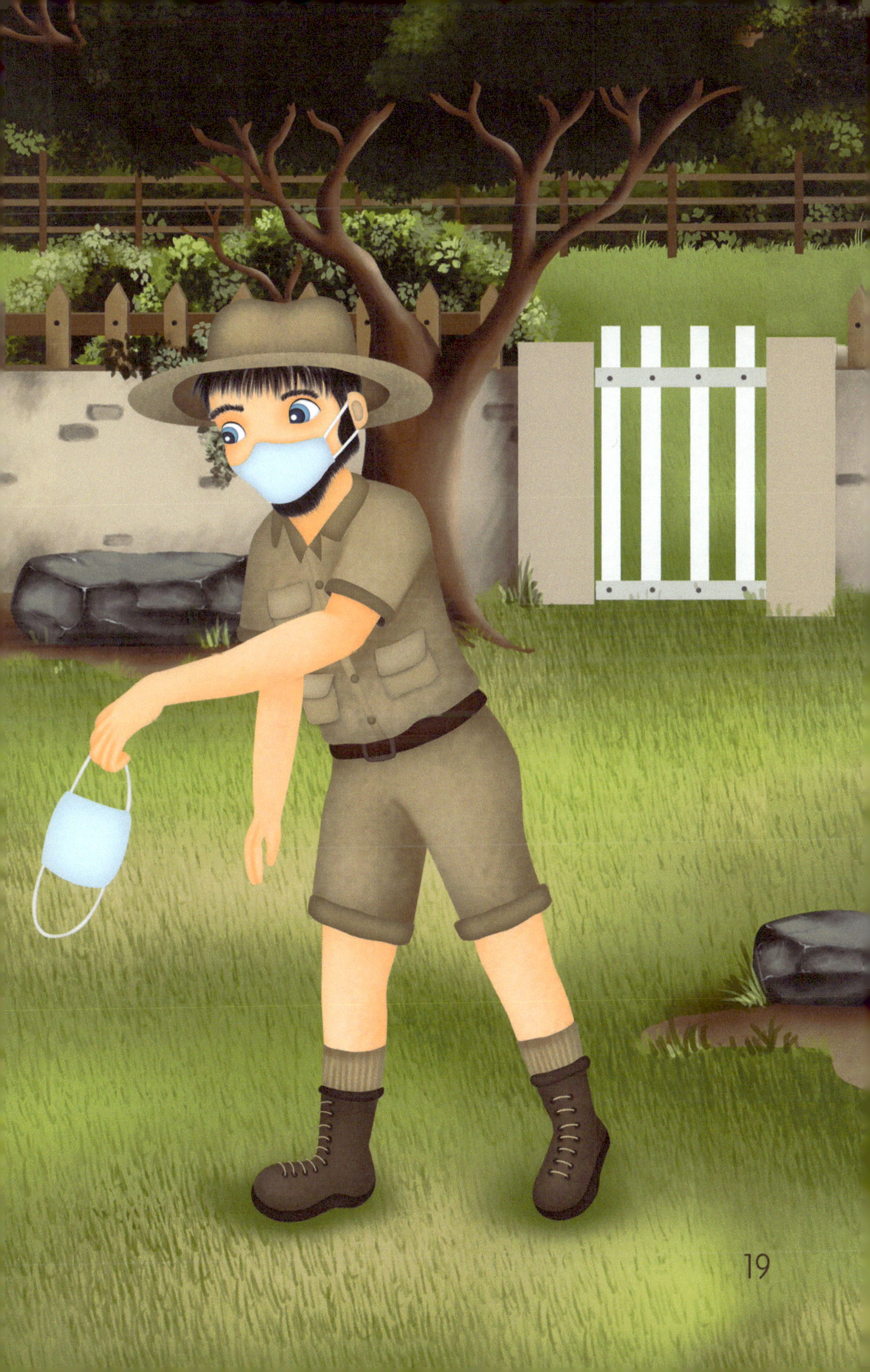

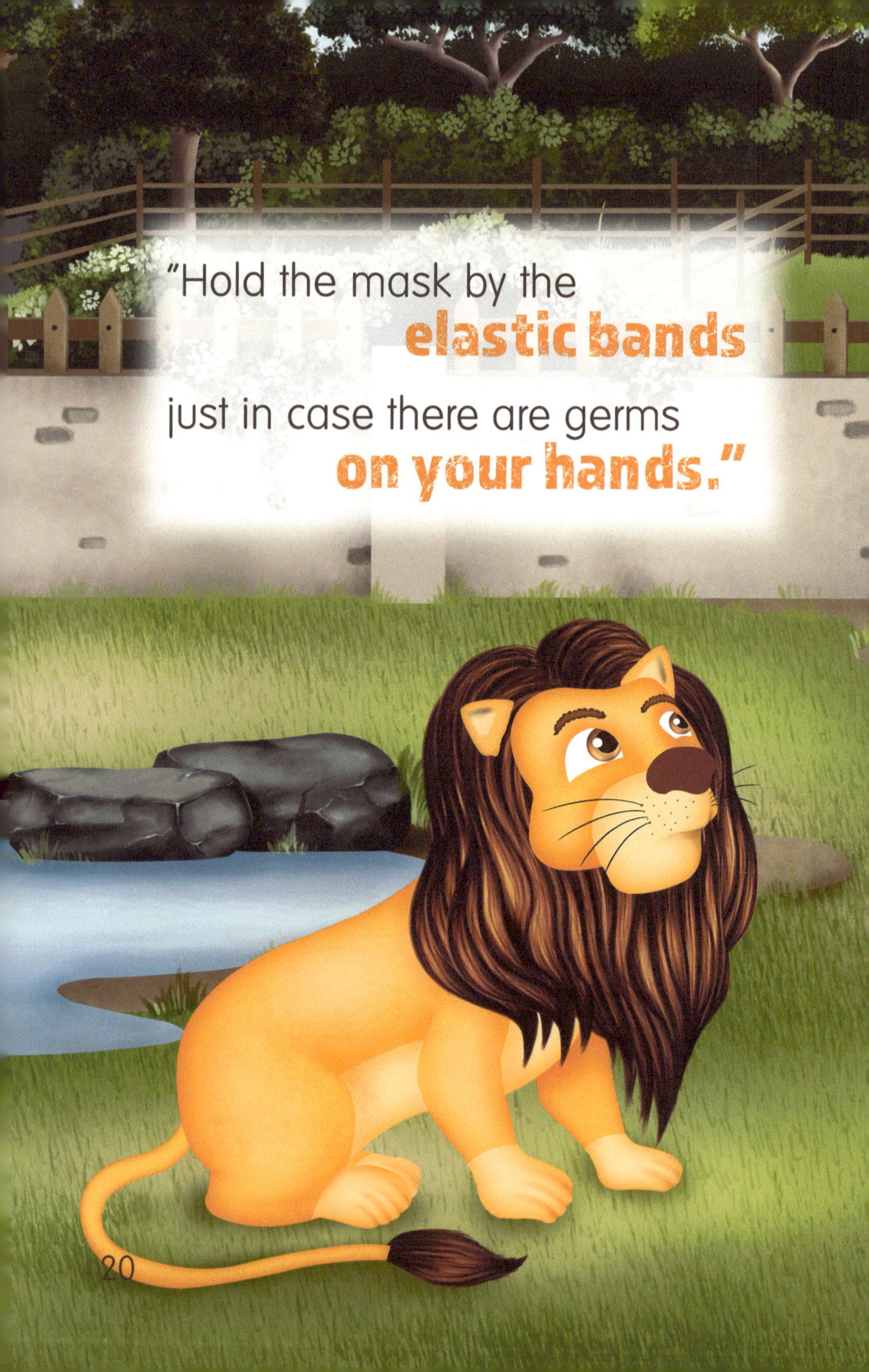

"Hold the mask by the elastic bands

just in case there are germs on your hands."

20

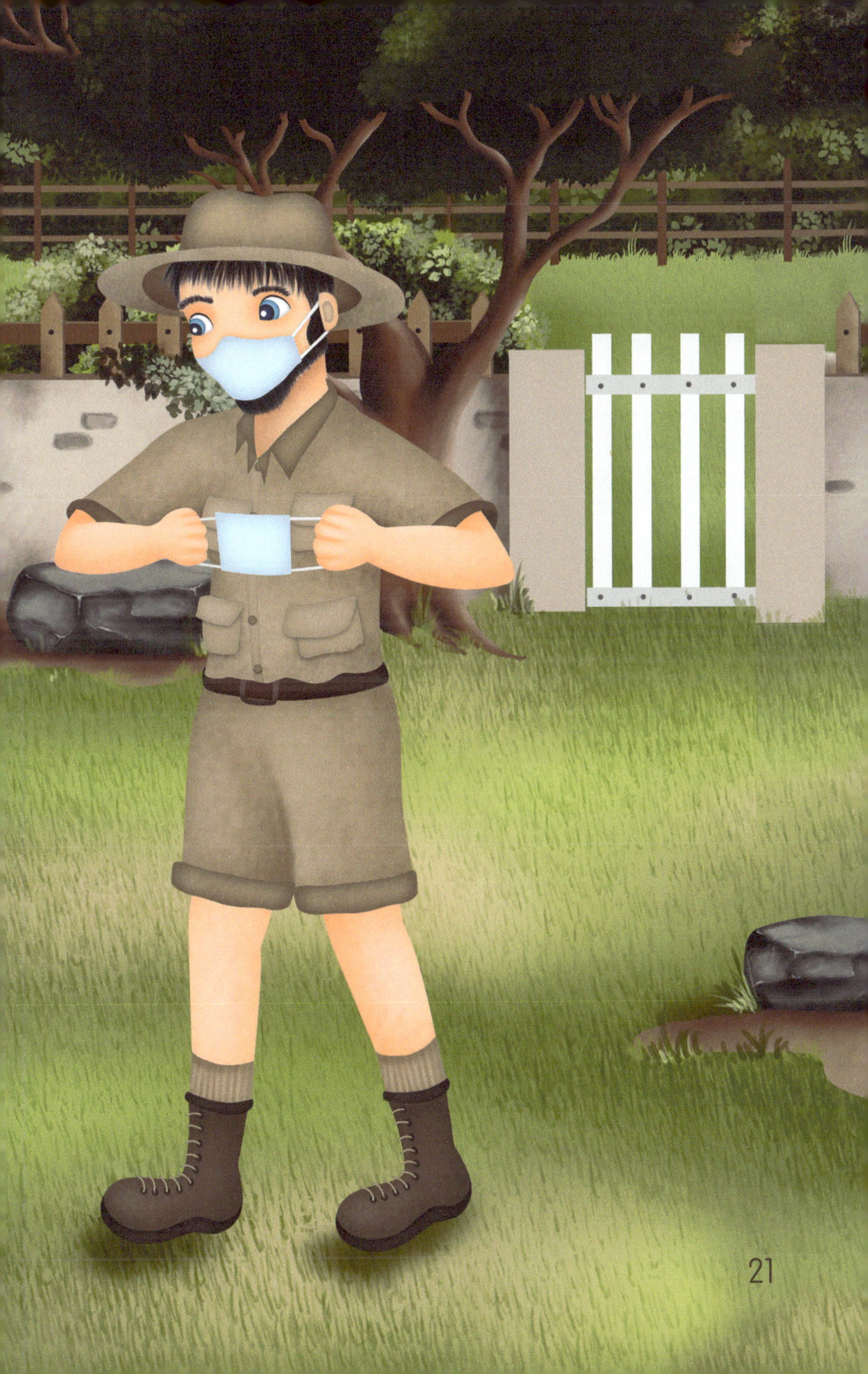

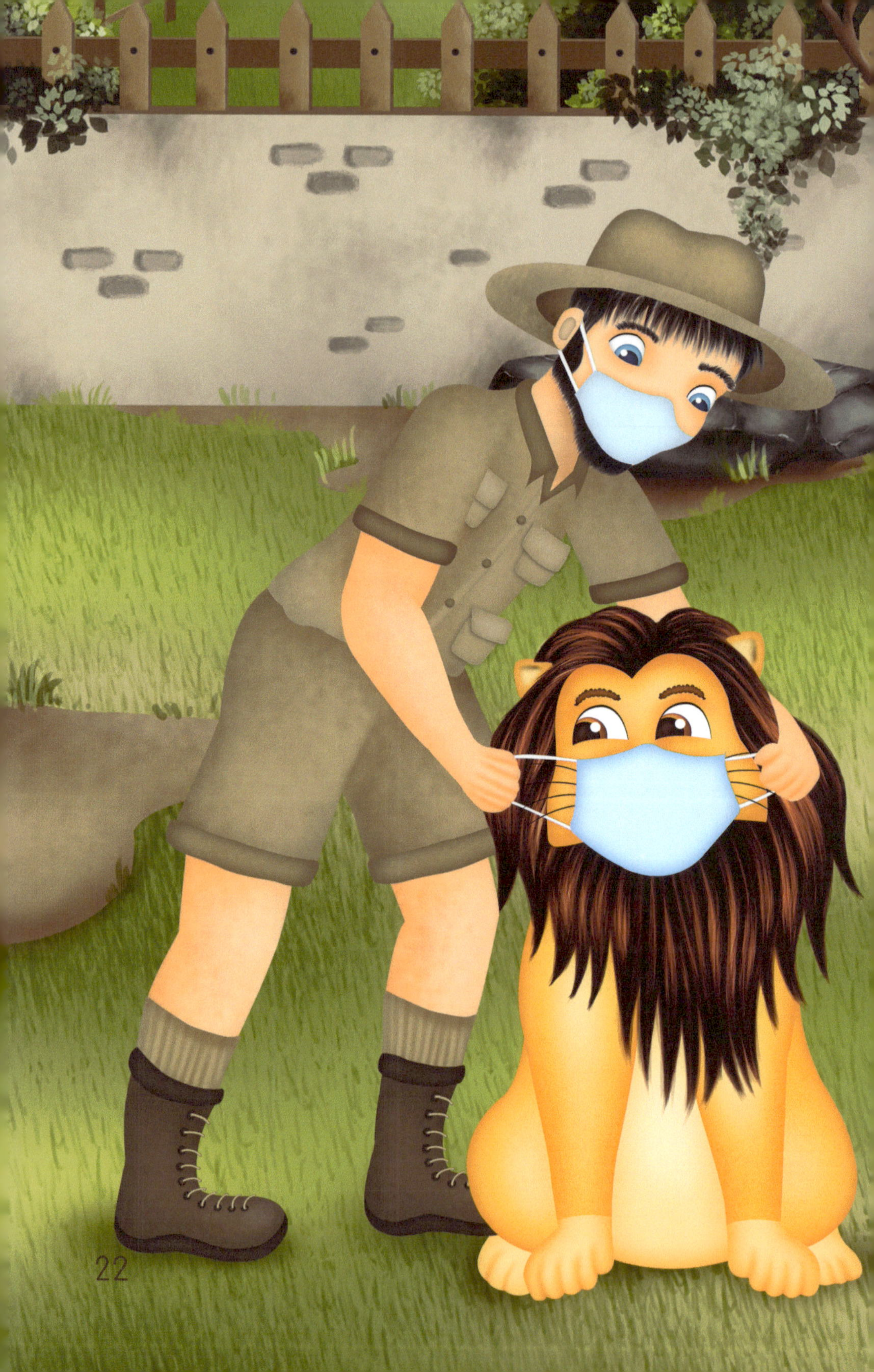
22

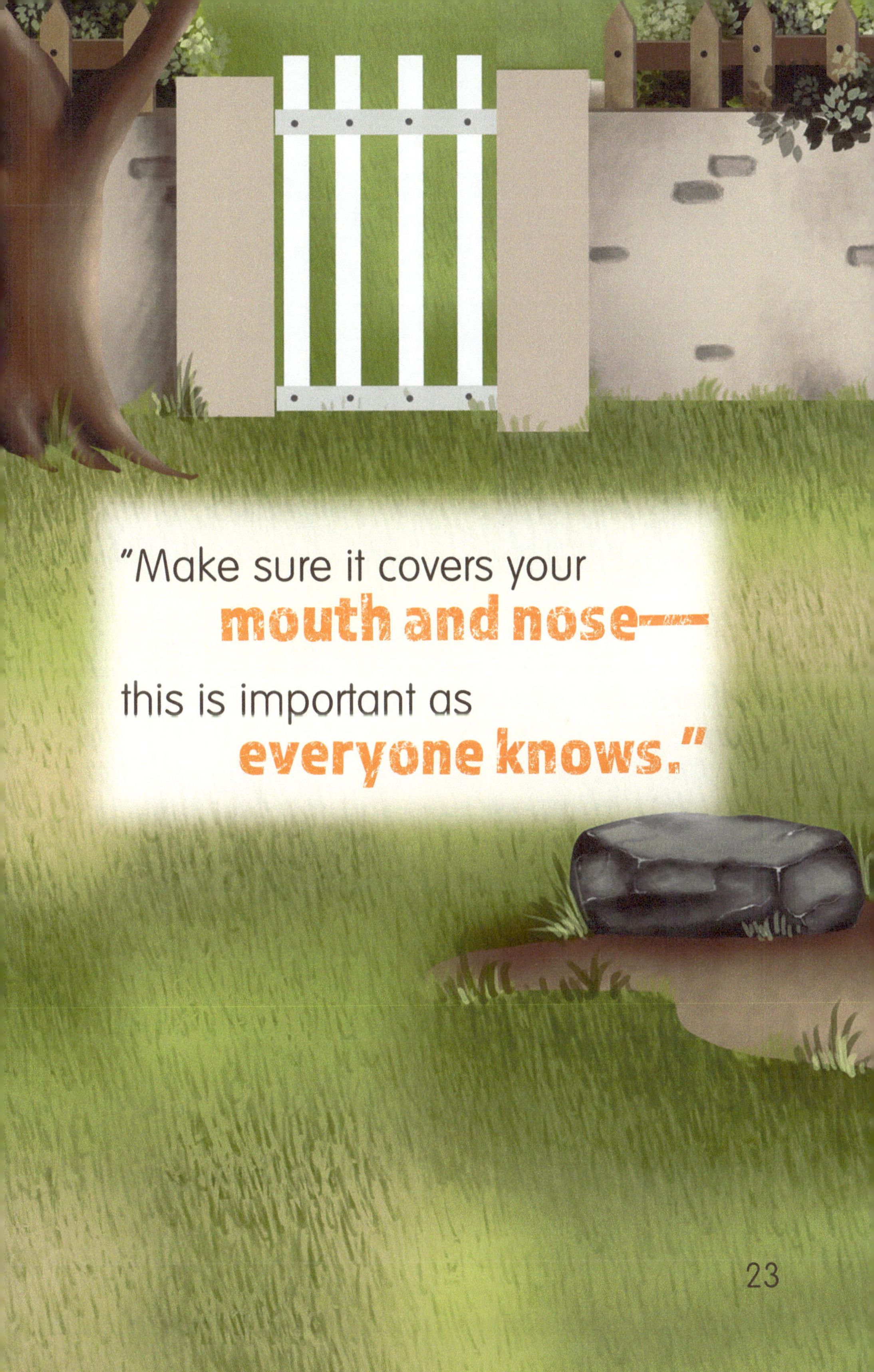
"Make sure it covers your
mouth and nose—
this is important as
everyone knows."

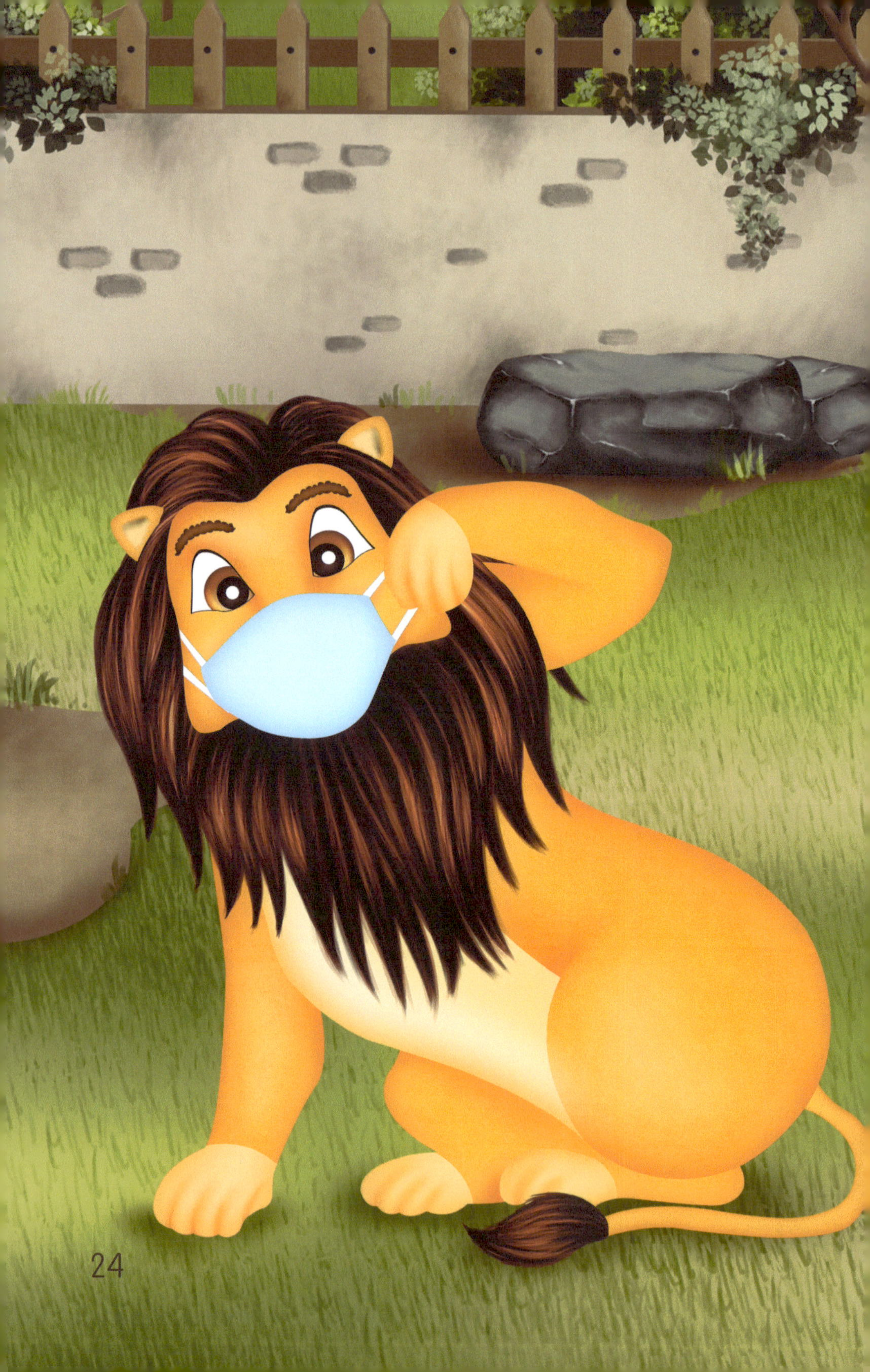

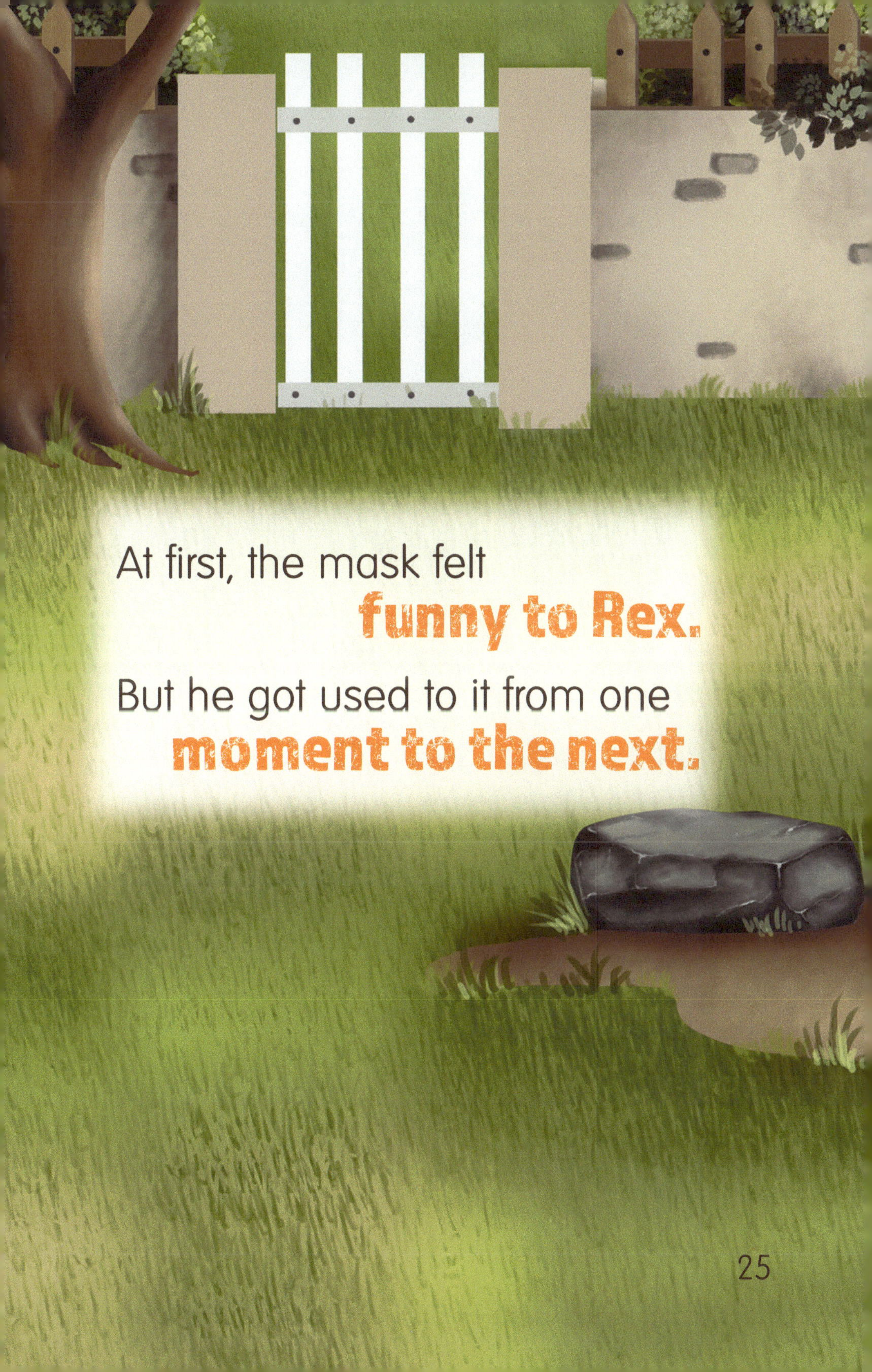

At first, the mask felt **funny to Rex.**

But he got used to it from one **moment to the next.**

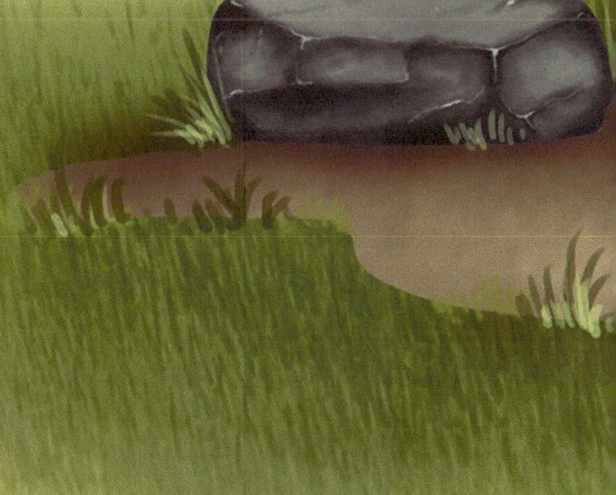

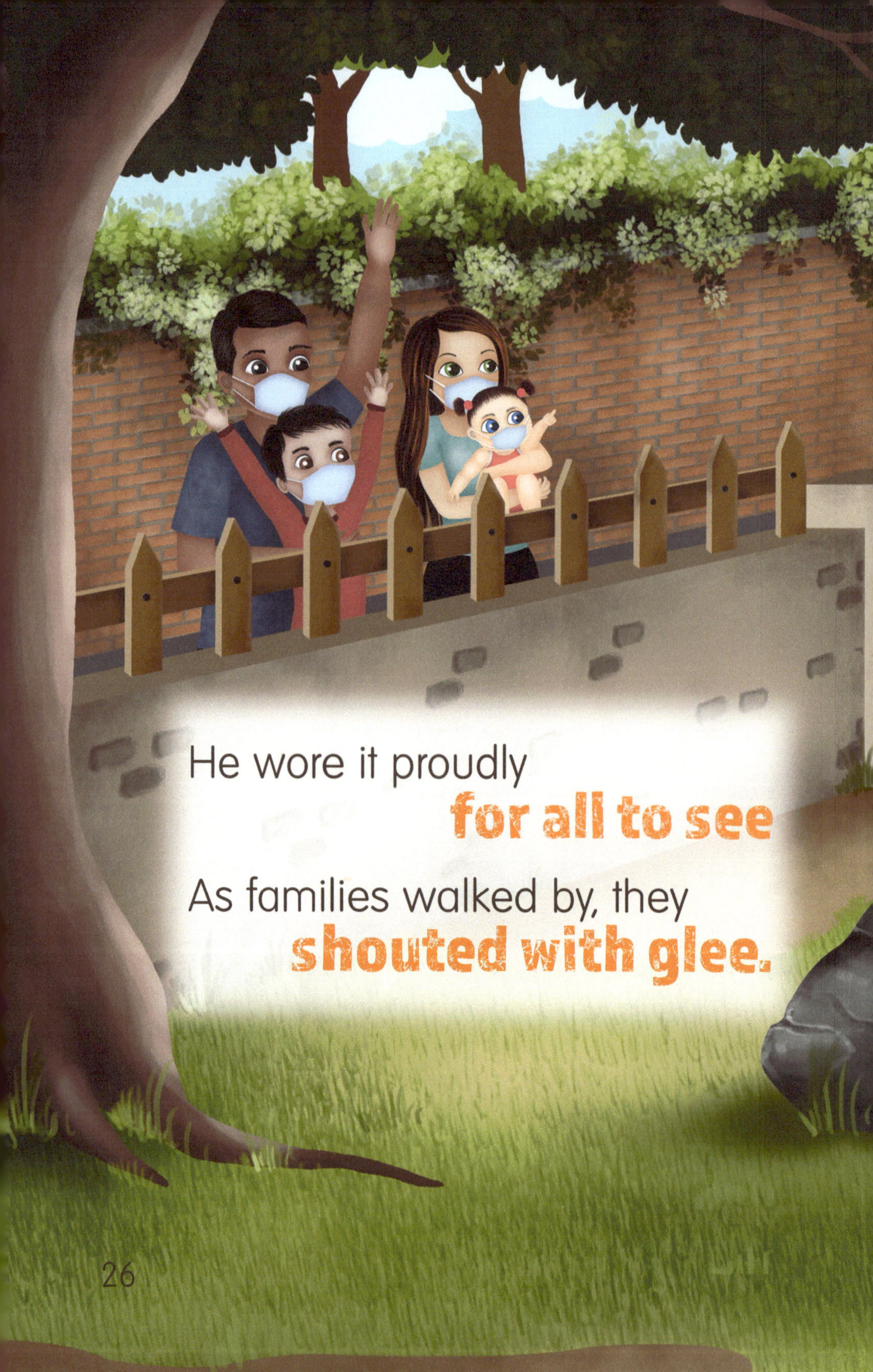

He wore it proudly
for all to see

As families walked by, they
shouted with glee.

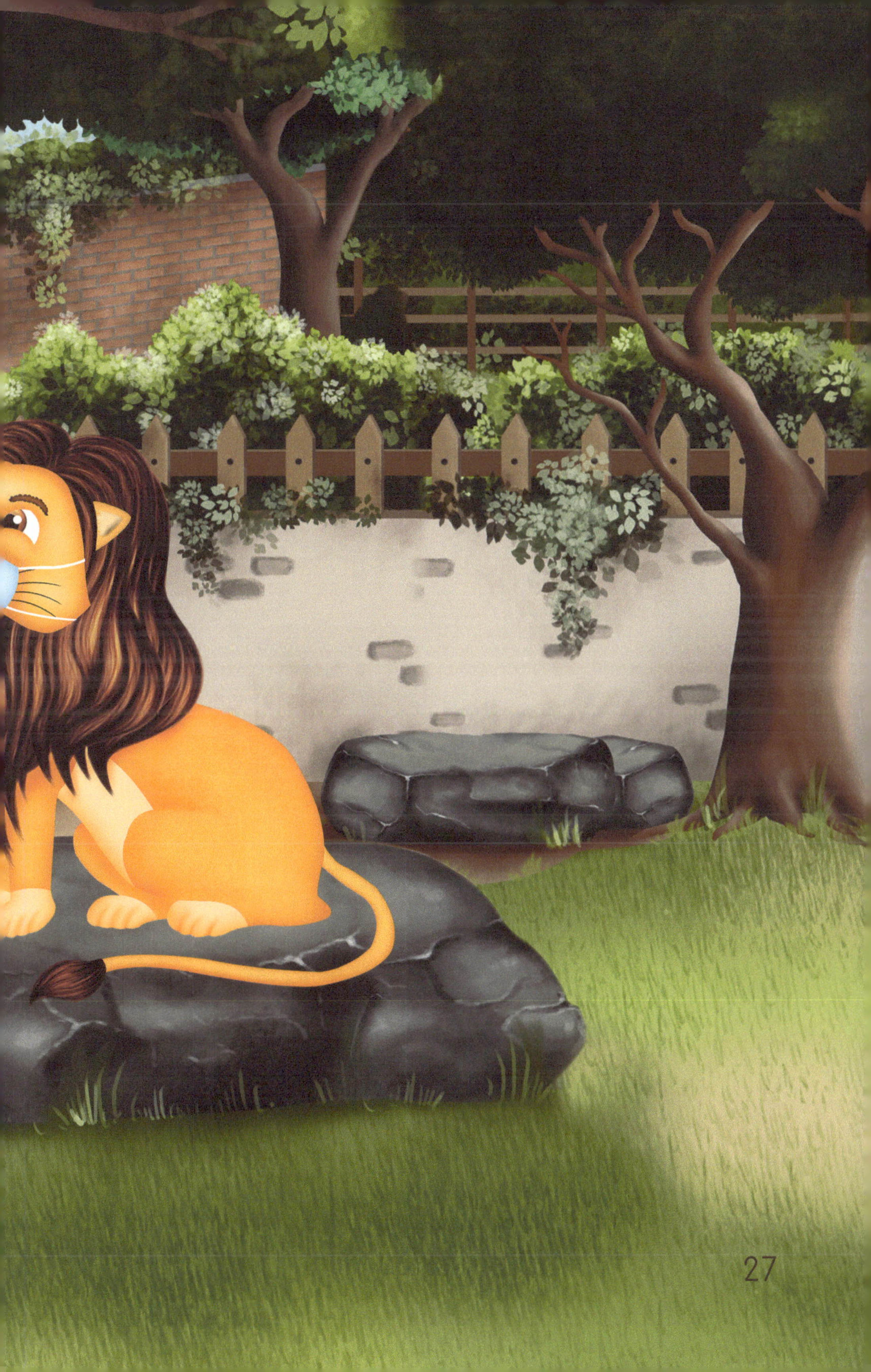

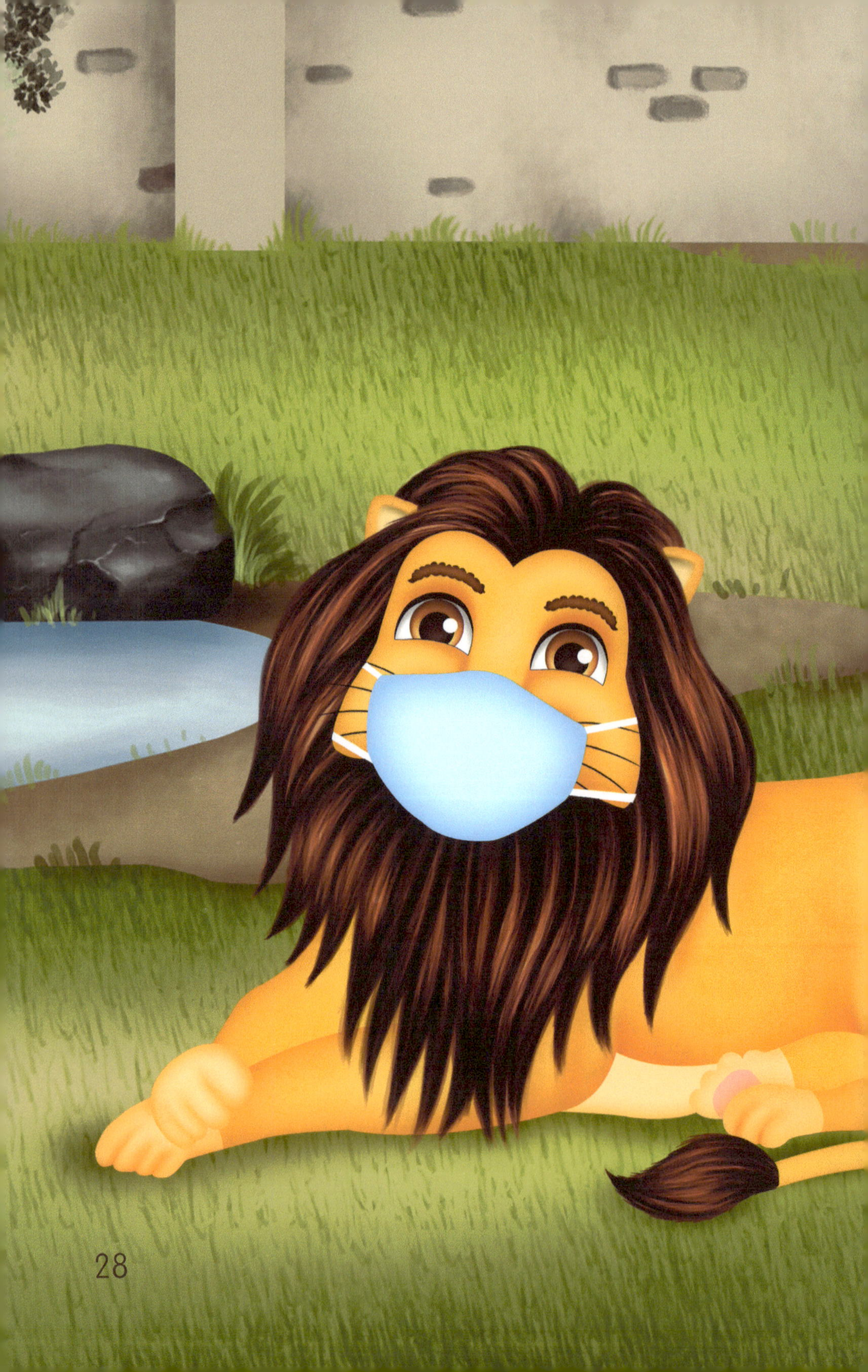

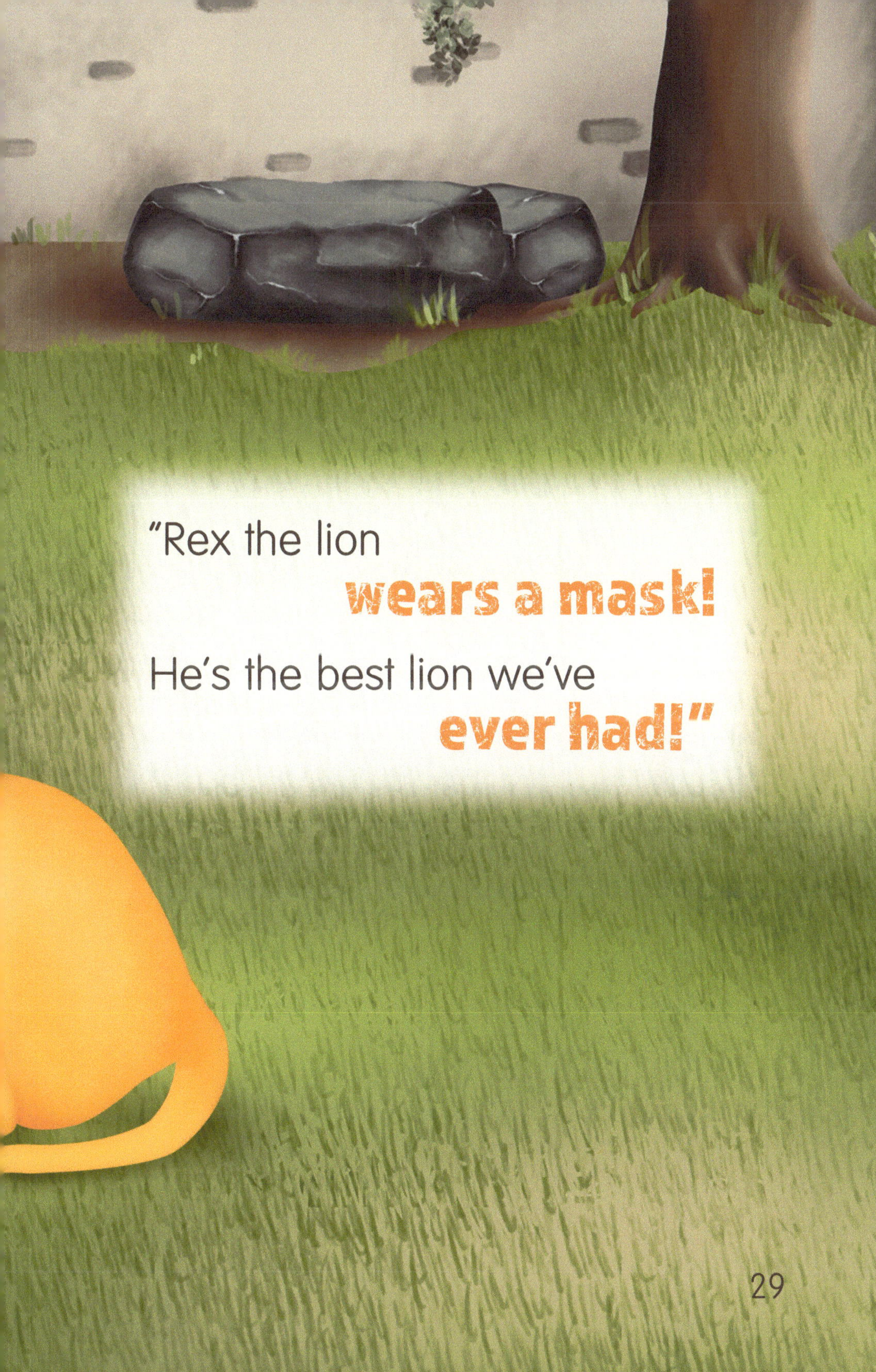

"Rex the lion wears a mask!
He's the best lion we've ever had!"

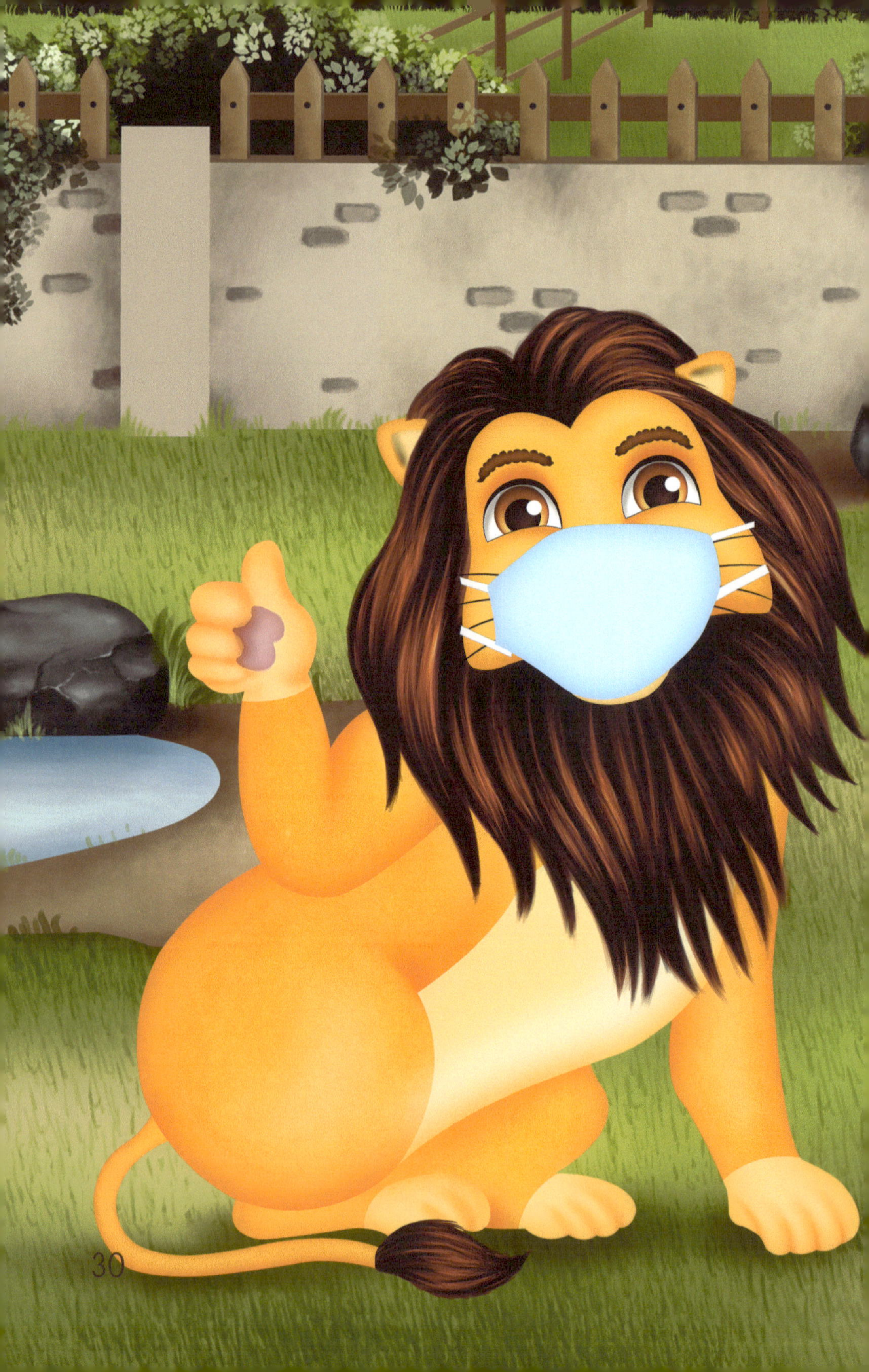

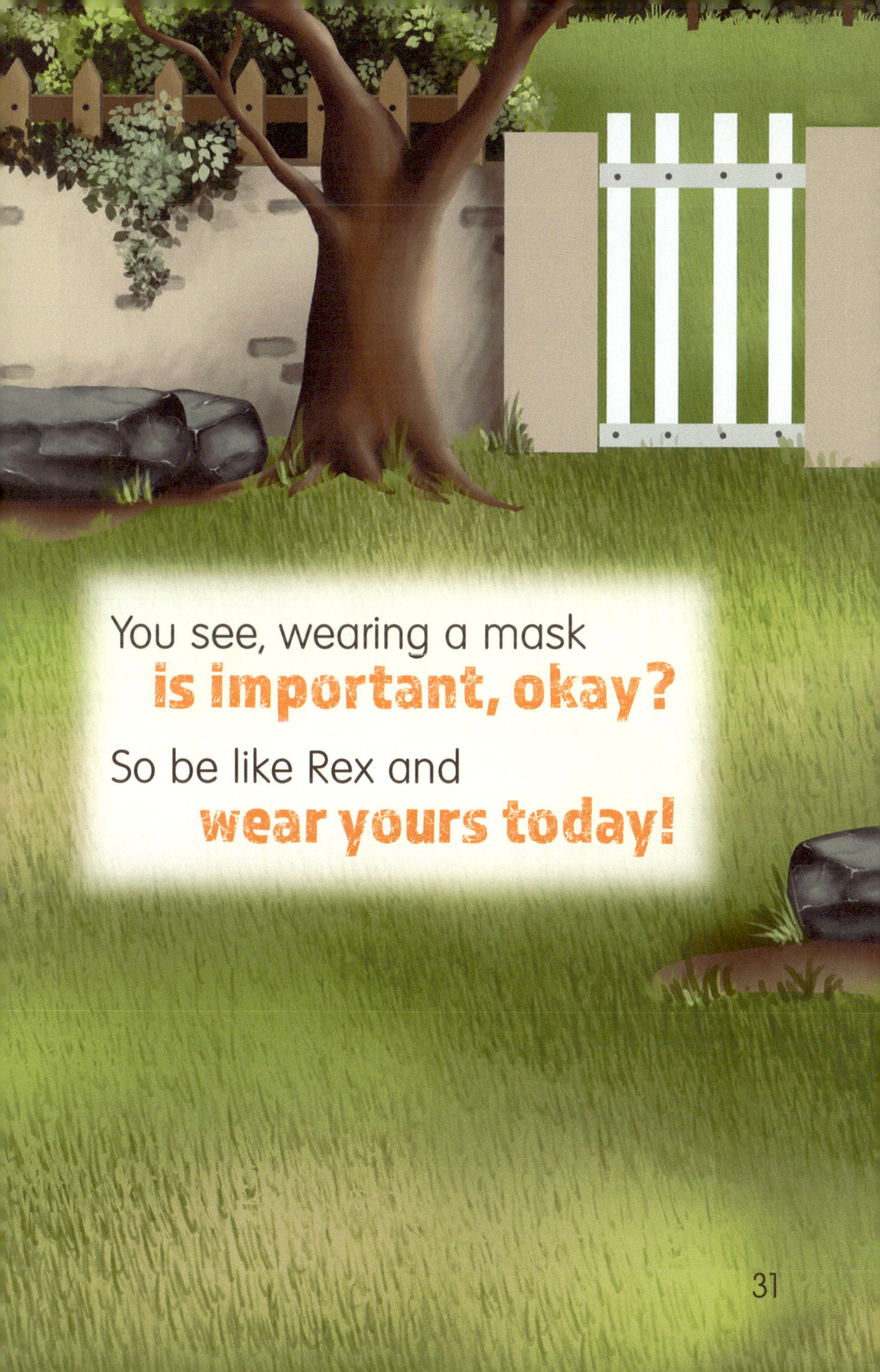

You see, wearing a mask
is important, okay?
So be like Rex and
wear yours today!

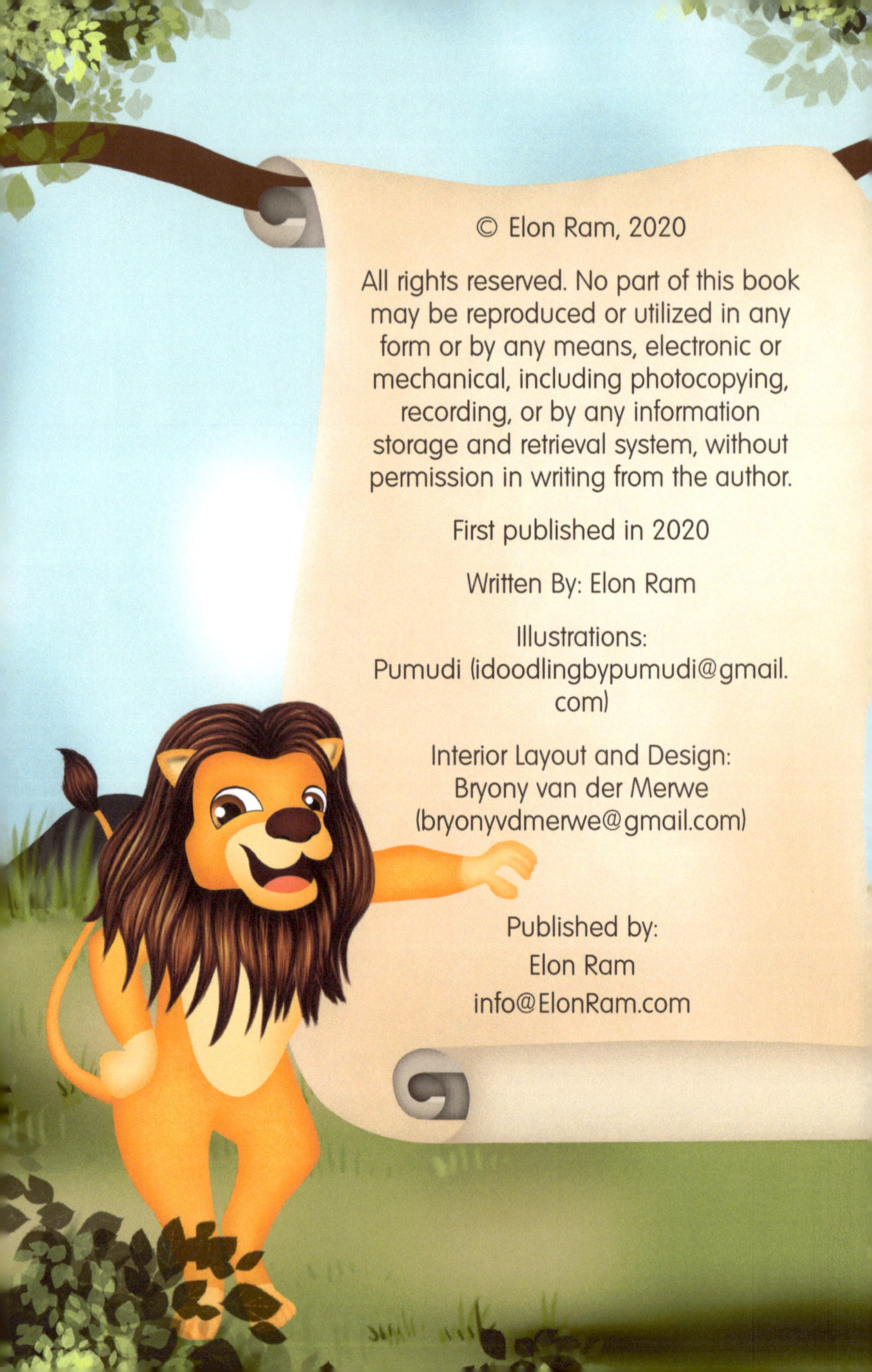

First published in 2020

Written By: Elon Ram

Illustrations:
Pumudi (idoodlingbypumudi@gmail.com)

Interior Layout and Design:
Bryony van der Merwe
(bryonyvdmerwe@gmail.com)

Published by:
Elon Ram
info@ElonRam.com